The Pink Purpose

My Story...For His Glory

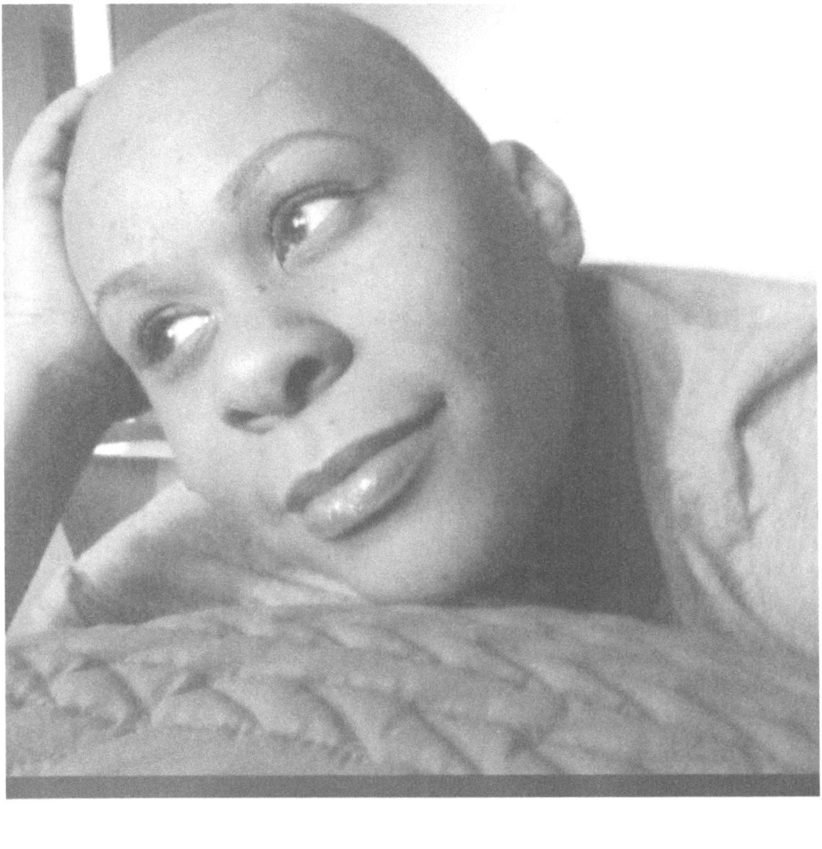

The Pink Purpose My Story…For His Glory

The Pink Purpose   My Story for His Glory

Published by the DancinWriter for

Suite 74 the Publishing Room

TITLE ID: 6501429

ISBN: 978-1537104232

ONLY with WRITTEN permission can any part of this book be reproduced for quotes, use of photos and or excerpts. This book may not be reproduced in partial or total without the exact permission of the author and publisher.

For any questions regarding our support group please contact us at

www.TheDancinWriter.com

dancinwriter@yahoo.com

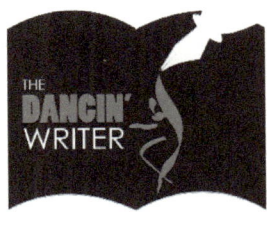 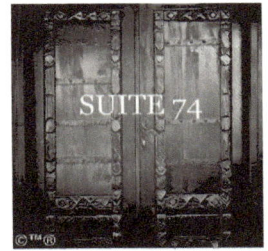

The Pink Purpose　　　　　　　　My Story for His Glory

I'm so thankful and blessed....

My Lord, my Savior, my healer, my deliverer, my Father and my friend; Jesus Christ.... It gets no better than living for and with you! I'm thankful for this thing called life. Every day with you, is sweeter than the day before! –your servant forever

My husband, my best friend, my Boogie, Ram... You loved me at my lowest point; called me beautiful when there was nothing but ashes to see. I laughed through my pain and cried 'til I felt joy again, always with you by my side. Your heart is priceless and for that I will protect it at ALL costs!!! I love you with every heartbeat, hug and steamed lobster tail! (you KNOW how I feel about my lobster tails! ☺Hugs and kisses forEVERs-your wife. *My sequel, my daughter, my pride and joy*, Iyliyah R.G. Young, You are magnificent proof of God's grace in my life. This journey tried to break us, but instead it fortified our bond. We are forever a team! (We've even gained three more teammates!) Remember to always reverence God. He's amazingly manifesting His power right before your eyes. Don't ever let the devil make you blink!-Love Mommy To my wedding gifts I get to open every day.... *Zaniah and Mahogany*, the love I have for you, it's immeasurable. Thank you for giving me not only the title 'bonus Mom' but loving me like I bore you! You are a joy to watch grow! I love you with everything in me! –Always, Mom2 *My mom*, THANK YOU! I've watched you lose a child, but not your faith. I've watched you suffer but never complain. When I think strength, I SEE you! I thank God for your praying spirit, your love, support AND patience with faith during my journey. God favored you and answered your prayers. We've been through a lot, but God proves himself to be in the midst every time and every trial. We owe him everything we are... and will ever be. Continue to live in your favor! We love and appreciate you! *Wallace*, my homie, the man I get to call on for everything a daddy's girl would...and he comes running... ...Thank you for all the fussing but still making sure I got to the hospital any time I had to call! Lol thank you for being protective and loving! You da best! *To my sisters, my prayer partners, my accountability, the Gina to my Pam and the Ethel to my Lucy, my girls….. NeNe*, we're family, but the friendship is so solid! Thank you for EVERYTHING! You already know what you mean to me can never be put into black and white. Heartbeats can't be written down! Love you girl! *Michele*, Thank you so much for believing real friends can come in later in life like they've been there all your life. Your strength during my weakest time, your quiet but POWERFUL spirit is second to none I love you. **NeNe & Michele.** You guys kept me level headed. You both understood texting over speaking it into the atmosphere. You held me together, even if it meant getting cut by the pieces of a broken me. I love you and your hubbies for lending y'all to me all the time! Thanks Estee, thanks Manny! And my **Chance!** You NEVER let me go hungry! Thank you for your private prayers and your texts, and just being my girl for life! Will always be the trio!!!! Love you for real! My pink sister who KEEPS me level headed throughout the work day, and keeps my laughter going long after it's done. *Zenobia,* we don't take the word 'friend' lightly. I will always have your back in prayer and in these streets ☺(Mall behavior! Insider) Thank you for showing me the real meaning of loyalty and light! Forever connected! ***My Bishop, Hezekiah Walker, Bishop Designate, Dr. Neil S. Harris, Elder-Elect Emanuewell Clay***, when the three of you prayed over me, I knew I would be okay…. If for nothing else, God came to see about me on your behalf. Thank you for every word spoken over the pulpit, the sidewalk, the café, the hallway…the phone… everywhere you had a chance, you spoke life into me. I'm honored to be a 'son'. I appreciate and love my leadership! My church, Love Fellowship Tabernacle, thank you for your strength! Lastly…My family, here's the hope and prayers manifested. Take heed. Do it again! Keep believing. Then, believe again! I love being connected by blood to yall! 285 FOREVER

      Always…… the Pink DancinWriter, Francys Renee

PREFACE

Hello. My name is Francys Renee and I am four years into my forever as a survivor. I am sharing this story with you for two reasons; to help someone who may be going through it, and to help someone who has come out of it.

There is something to be said about living after cancer.... but we can't speak on that until we can speak about living before it, and with it. Life changes when it faces death. What was important doesn't seem to be anymore.... and what wasn't important seems to become the very air you breathe. I am a faith walker. A Christ believing, Bible confessing, all things are possible if you believe survivor who, truthfully, was sick. I was sick. I am now healed. I am in good health... mentally, physically and spiritually. Those are my daily confessions and I wanted to share them with you.

There is someone reading this that needs to say that out loud. You are healed. You are in good health... mentally, physically and spiritually. Even if you can't say it right now, I'm praying that by the end of my story..... It will be the beginning of yours and of His glory in your life.

If you are sick in your body, I am praying that it never makes its way to your heart or your mind. Believe in your heart and command your mind to speak to your body. It was created to be in good health, not my words but God's. Don't believe me? God's word confirms it.... *"Beloved, I pray that you may prosper in all things and be in health, just as your soul prospers"* **3.John 1:2**. This book is dedicated to every cancer patient, every breast cancer survivor, and every fighter who is now resting in glory. With God, all things are possible. Strength over weakness, peace over chaos, love over hurt, and LIFE over death! I'm humbled by my journey.

God's will for my life is my desire. My story is… for His Glory.

> *"...this sickness is not unto death, but for the glory of God that the Son of God might be glorified thereby"*

John 11:4

DESTINY OVER DIAGNOSIS

May of 2011. Like any other day off, I was home cleaning and repositioning things in my house. I was moving a little too quickly and fell into a stack of boxes filled with my books. I hit my left breast on the box pretty hard and it responded to the hit quickly. The swelling and the pain was almost unbearable.

Thinking it was just a regular injury, I waited until the next day to call my doctor. That morning, the breast was hard and hot to the touch. At that time in my life, I wasn't familiar with the signs of cancer because it never directly affected my life enough for me to become knowledgeable. I did however know something was off. I knew something was wrong.

I went to my internist who looked at my left breast that nearly doubled in size over night and she immediately sent me to a breast specialist. After just looking at me externally, she was certain what was going on internally. She advised me of what it looked like. It was unfortunately that word I had heard over television commercials, walking past that "section" in the hospital, hearing it in the mouths of other people and about other *older* family members but never directly to me. Cancer.

Cancer?

Yes. Cancer.

How could *that* be? All I did was fall into some boxes. How did a trip get me here? How was I was being sent to a specialist to confirm a disease? Were you now able to catch a disease from falling? I was too confused.

Dr. Lori Cohen, my internist for over a decade and I had developed a certain level of comfort with her. She had a way as a doctor that that made all of her patients feel like they were being treated by their old friend. She made you feel safe and made trusting her an easy thing. It came naturally to heed to her instructions because she always remained fair and objective and made sure you understood that each person case was a different case.

From sitting in the waiting room with other patients, you talk, and you learned that you all have the same opinion about the doctor who you usually had to wait a little longer for because she took her time with each of her patients on her roster which seemed pretty long.

So even though this was a very different time in my life and I was so confused, it was nothing for me to listen to her instructions and go to the doctor. I trusted her judgment and those she referred me to. I was even impressed I was able to see the doctor she referred to me the same day. At the same time I was a little nervous at the urgency Dr. Cohen had.

It was that day, in that referred office, with that referred doctor that I would learn quickly; every doctor wasn't as compassionate as the next. It didn't matter that you were alone, and afraid. They didn't all possess kind bed side manner either.

This was the doctor that performed the first biopsy on my breast; the one that confirmed my internists' suspicions.

You would think I would never forget her name or her face. As I write this and try my best to recall it, all I can remember is that she was an older woman and had blonde hair. I remember her office being dark and cold and sad. I remember feeling dreary when I walked in and empty when I walked out. I remember the exact moment and every detail after walking out of the office and the door closing behind me. The water fountain to my right, the man talking on his cell phone to my left, he had on a blue suit, black glasses and was upset he had to end his lunch early. However, I cannot place the receptionist, the nurse or the doctor. All I remember was how she made me feel.

It may sound weird to make such a note of that but as I explain; I hope it makes more sense. I walked in to her office and it was cold. White everything.....no decor, just clinic looking. Her first words to me were "This looks like cancer." It wasn't "hello, how are you? How did this happen? What happened?"

Nothing.

She looked at me with such sorrow on her face... and she said "When I put this needle in your breast, if I don't get any fluid, that's not good" She started talking about all of these symptoms and what they derived from. I didn't understand a thing she was saying. I was alone, and afraid, because all the terminologies she was using was not 'patient friendly'. I was so mad and so scared at the same time.

Once she pulled the needle out, there wasn't any fluid.

She shook her head and told me I could get dress and she would call me with the final results. I got dressed and walked out. I didn't make it past the lobby before I started to cry. Fear set in hard. During this time I was dating a guy I really liked so I instinctively called him first to tell him about my day. His response didn't help. He told me that we needed to stop speaking because he cared about me a lot and didn't want to watch me die. Really? That call did more damage. It took me a while to stop being mad at him. I realize... only those who know better do better and speak better. If you don't know what to say... ignorance quickly speaks for you. I don't blame him at all. Not now anyway. Not anymore. I blame myself because I trusted the instinct of my flesh and in return I received flesh, and we all know flesh will fail you every time.

There is always a need to have a plan of action when you are going through something. Just like you have the IN CASE OF AN EMERGENCY numbers to call on your fridge or wallet? You need to have that in your phone to call when you're in trouble also. Everyone is not going to deposit the right things in your ear at the most crucial time. You must have a plan. Have your prayer warriors on speed dial! I diverted from my plan, and it delayed a much needed deposit in my life.

After the longest day imaginable, I finally got home and I called my 'sister friends'. After I told them what happened, they vowed to seek the face of the Lord for me and told me to do the same thing.

We called the devil a liar... spoke that I was not going to deal with cancer in my body.

We were going to war!

We had the right response.

However, three days later, my results came back. There was a cancerous tumor found in my breast.

Wait. What? Didn't I pray? Didn't we turn down our plates? Isn't that what the Word told us to do? Call things that are not as though they were? What happened here? What did I miss?

You wouldn't believe me if I told you right here.... So you're just going to have to keep reading. Because I promise you, if you're in fear right now, you've missed it too.

Dealing with the diagnosis, I had to make a plan. I needed to figure out my next step. I have an aunt, who even though she is now retired, she will always be the 'family nurse'. We call her for everything from a common cold, to well, a cancer diagnosis. I remember calling her and telling her about my horrible visit and my results. I cried on the phone because I didn't understand, I spoke that I didn't have cancer, I prayed, I fasted and I believed, but the test still came back positive for cancerous growth. My aunt was gentle on the phone yet full of authority and kind at the same time.

After hearing my story about my terrible experience, she advised me to seek a second opinion. She gave me the number to Memorial Sloan Kettering and instructed me to call as soon as we hung up because the hospital is very busy and it may take long to get an appointment, and with my breast steadily growing, time was not something we had to waste.

I called Memorial Sloan almost immediately, looking for the doctor she suggested. The doctor she suggested wasn't available, but Dr. Heather McArthur was and she could see me as soon as the following Thursday. I secured my appointment and called my girlfriend up, asked if she would come with me because I knew better this time than to go alone. I wanted a support system. I didn't expect the worse, but I prepared for anything.

Because this particular section of the book is about just the diagnosis, I won't get into much that designed that day for my destiny as of yet...but I will touch on the difference I experienced. When I walked into the Evelyn Lauder Breast Cancer Center, I was greeted with smiles and warmth as if they were already silently cheering for me. They didn't know me, I didn't know them, but we all had a common enemy, cancer. Because this place particularly focused on the cancer of the breast, they knew that somehow I was directly connected with it and I guess they wanted me to know I was in a good place.

When we walked in, my future oncologist' receptionist was so kind. Her name was Michelle. My girlfriend and I laughed because everybody talked and smiled the same. We almost thought they were trained to all speak and smile the same way. Everybody was just so nice.

When I met my oncologist, I saw strength. I saw assurance and I saw hope. She smiled at me, and welcomed me into her office. I felt differently immediately. I got real confident... like... yes *she* knows what *she's* doing. She knows what to look for; I'm sure the other place made a mistake so *she* will tell me I'm fine. Another biopsy and CT scan later proved me wrong again.

June 2011 I was officially diagnosed with *Local Advanced Breast Cancer*.

The cancer found in the left breast was dormant for years, but never moved....that's what made it local. The size of the tumor was one of a grapefruit. That's what made it advanced. I was afraid, but with my friend there speaking the right things, like "God got you and He got this. You're gonna be alright friend! God is a healer friend! Watch Him do it" I began to feel like a champion but I didn't even win yet. I will forever love Michele Clay for her support, her friendship, but most of all, her faith and prayer life.

I didn't know what my purpose was in this and I hadn't made the distinguished understanding yet whether or not this was a sickness my sin brought on and I was being punished or was this part of my destiny in His design for His glory to be shown through my life that had nothing to do with my past but everything to do with my future.

More often than not, when people see others afflicted, they immediately think that they are being punished by God for sin.

It is true and biblical that deeds done in the body you have to answer for….however… I don't believe every answer is an affliction. There are punishments, and then there are consequences. God doesn't work like that. There is no sickness in Him. And IN HIM I move and have my being so…… it didn't come from Him. Does he allow it? Sure. We bring things on ourselves by not eating the right thing, engaging in promiscuous activity, living beyond the hedge of protection, and living out of disobedience, overweight, underweight and so on and so on. In my case, I was diagnosed just as I was living and doing the right thing. I had decided earlier in that year that I was fully committed to the life of salvation. Praying, fasting, speaking and living the word. Funny thought occurred to me.

When I was sinning, I was just as healthy. I didn't have a nary a cold that lasted more than a day or two. And now, when I completely gave my will over to God, I'm diagnosed with cancer.

At least that would be how the devil wanted me to look at it. God did it. He made me sick because He was mad at me. No. Wrong. So wrong. Here's the truth, well my truth for my life anyway.

God allowed the devil to touch my body because God knew He could trust me with it, even if I didn't think I could handle it. God knew I could and would handle it for His glory.

He knew He could trust me to walk in the room sick in my body still speaking His glory to those who might not hear it any other time. He knew that someone was watching and needed to see His healing power manifested on earth. He knew that I would make it through and I would write his book. I would let the world know, that the diagnosis was part of my destiny to be the epistle you see before you.

I am here declaring the works and THE WORD of the Lord. HE IS A HEALING GOD! Ask me how I know! I've seen Him do it! He allowed me to become weak, because His grace was sufficient and His power made perfect in my weakness. I believe that He waited, like a gentlemen, for me to get myself together. He waited until I was committed to His voice so that the devil didn't have any chance at getting any glory from this. He waited until I was ready. J.J. Hairston said it best... it PUSHED ME into my destiny. God knew it would make me who He called me to be!!! With that being said, I will end this chapter with the lyrics to the song I listen to everyday sometimes all day! My diagnosis pushed me into my destiny! Thank you JJ for this song… it is my anthem..

"God gave me a vision of where I would be, but he didn't show me what I'd go through on the journey; But everything that I faced prepared me for what God has for me to do. So now that I'm here, I can praise Him for all I that had to go through. What the devil meant for evil, God used to get the glory. 'cause it pushed me into my... It pushed me into my destiny. God used it to make me who He called me to be. All of the tests and trials were a part of God's plan; they have all made me stronger, and taught me how to trust Him. That's why my praise is so crazy, And often misunderstood; 'cause what the enemy thought would destroy me, God turned it around for my good. What the devil meant for evil, God used to get the glory. 'cause it pushed me into my... It pushed me into my destiny. God used it to make me who He called me to be. All the trouble, all the pain brought me closer to Him. It was good that I was afflicted, 'cause it made me who I am! It pushed me into my………… it pushed me into my destiny! Thank you for pushing me... Thank you for pushing me... yeah! 'cause every struggle (It pushed me) and that sickness (It pushed me) The nights I cried (It pushed me) And that pain (It pushed me) Thought it would take me out (It pushed me) But it pushed me further! (It pushed me) Now I can say (Now I... can... say!) Thank you for pushing me Thank you for pushing me... yeah. God used it to make me Who He called me to be

chapter 1

"Choosing Faith over Fear"

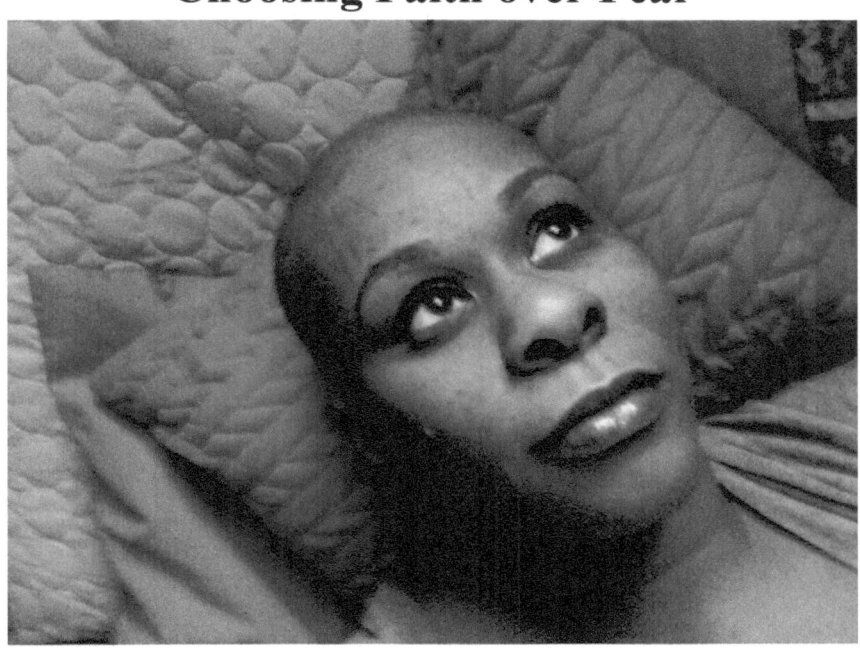

"For God has not given us a spirit of fear, but of power and of love and of sound mind"
2 Timothy 1:7 NKJV

A cancer diagnosis can be scary, for unbelievers *and* believers alike. That moment, when a doctor tells you that you have a deadly disease, that precise second, you have to decide how your entire journey will go from that point. You have to decide whether to remain fearful, or faithFULL! What I mean by faithFULL is FULL OF FAITH! So full of it, that there is no room for fear.

As I sat in my oncologist office with my sister friend Michele Clay, I thought to myself…what am I going to do? Am I going to believe and move on, or be afraid? I figured, since I've believed GOD this long; why not go the whole way. I've been singing about His powers, HEARING about His wonders, and speaking His deliverance I was now at the stage where nothing that I would say from this point on would be second hand or hearsay.

Everything I spoke about would be something I myself witnessed; within myself.

He is a healer, and I would know it for myself.
He is a keeper, and I would know that for myself.
He is a way maker, and I would know it for myself.

All I could do was pray. I prayed hard and I prayed faithfully. If you ever want to hear a good prayer, listen to someone who's experiencing some trouble.

I was facing a fear unlike any other and I had to be honest about it. These doctors were telling me I had locally advanced breast cancer, which was the leading disease that African American women in their early to late thirties died from. What? Lord HELP! I prayed even in that oncologist office. I had to keep professing "Lord, I still believe." I had to convince myself.

As the doctor discussed the plan of action to beat my disease, I sat and I heard her. I never listened, I just heard. I am not deaf, so of course I heard her, but I am not dumb, therefore I did not listen. I did not receive her report. I still believed the report of the Lord; By His stripes…

So as I left the office, I made my necessary phone calls and told my family and close friends to tell them what that the doctor diagnosed me with breast cancer.

I never once allowed my mouth to say "I have breast cancer". When anyone asked me what was going on, I would say "The doctors said…"

I would not confess to having that disease. I knew the power of the tongue and life and death lies in it…So I chose the use of my power very carefully. Anyone who knows me knows my mouth is powerful!

So, from this point on, my mouth would speak nothing but life. I had made the decision and chosen my faith over any fear. I had chosen to believe the GOD I served! He said He was a healer and now I needed Him to show ME! He said that He would be my strength, He needed to SHOW me. I sat back and gave GOD the platform to be GOD. I chose my faith, and decided that nothing or no one would change my mind. There was no way that GOD would say a thing and not perform a thing. So, here goes Jesus…..fear overboard, faith in full motion.

The summer of 2011 would change my life forever. I had met one of the sweetest oncologists by the name of Dr. Heather McArthur, who had just returned from maternity leave when I arrived at Memorial Sloan Kettering. I had done my research on her, and she came with stellar written recommendations, awards, citations, and plain ol' 'thank yous' from previous and current patients. However, meeting her in person and experiencing her bedside manner was comforting.

She explained to me that the size of my tumor was very large, but 'we' were going to shrink it. That was it. She had too decided to have faith *with* me.
"When two or three are gathered...I will be in the midst....."

My tumor was extremely large and began to concern me because it started to grow which meant to me, that the cancer was spreading or gaining strength. But GOD! God's word and promises are so awesome. Just as quick as wrong thought would come I'm thankful that a scripture followed. The Word of God began to jump out of the book to me.
"Cast down imagination & every high thing that exalts itself against the knowledge of God" 2 Corinthians 10:5.

I had to bring my mind under subjection daily because the slightest words or concerns could break me.
Had I succumb to my own thoughts, I would not be here writing this testimonial.
As God would have it, it turned out that my thought or perhaps fearful and faithless reasoning was wrong...but let me not jump ahead! It's just hard not to write about where I came from, and not jump ahead fast knowing where I stand today.

My tumor had grown to the point where I couldn't wear regular bras anymore. One breast was a DD cup and the other had grown to a triple D almost E. It was that swollen.

My doctor was concerned about the cancer having travelled to my lymph nodes, which would mean the cancer had found its way into my blood stream. That would be an entire different outlook.

She had felt under my arm and it seemed as though I had a little inflammation under there, so she just did a worse case scenario and decided that she would treat the lymph nodes as though they were cancerous. So glad GOD is not like man. He never gives a worst case scenario!

As the visit went on, I remember asking a bunch of questions and one of them was "If the medicine works and it starts shrinking can I stop taking chemo?"

My doctor stopped me and said *"When* the medicine works…"

I smiled. GOD had sent me the right doctor who had the right speech!

She believed GOD whether she would admit it to me or not. You see, in that type of setting, religion was a touchy thing.

You weren't necessarily allowed to proclaim your belief. Weird thing though, there were chapels to pray. It was almost like; they knew there was a GOD, but which one you prayed to was totally up to you.

I saw it in my doctor's eyes though. Believers recognize believers! As we talked further in what would take place, she informed me that I had to complete my course of medication no matter how my response was great or less than great.

After a final look at all of my pathology reports, blood tests, mammograms, sonograms, CT scans, PET scans, biopsy results and all written reports accompanied by various pictures, my doctor had started the ball rolling on my fight with faith

I cannot seem to mention it enough.
I had an enormous tumor that had seemed to be in my body for a long time, but what Dr. McArthur couldn't understand is, that it hadn't metastasized, which means, it hadn't spread to any other organ. It remained in my breast tissue.

GOD had already started to show His hand in my situation. When I tell the story, I would always say "I would like to believe God said, that's it devil. You got from right here to right there. You can't move anywhere, and you can't involve anything else. This is all you got" Like, Jesus drew a line in the sand!

Dr. McArthur sat there looking at the images and with her hand on her cheek, looking at the images over her glasses, she kept saying

"I don't understand why it didn't move, or how it didn't, but Thank God it didn't"

I don't know if she had said "thank God" as a cliché phrase, but I said it, Michele said it and we all looked at each other, nodded our heads and moved from there. Once she got over the initial explanation, she sat back at her desk and looked at me for a minute before she spoke. She took a deep breath and questioned me.

"Are you okay?"

"I am fine" was my response; speaking it into the atmosphere. I would have to admit, I was a little nervous, but all the more ready to get the process started. My doctor looked at me, and then she looked back at her paper.

As she began to discuss what my chemotherapy would entail, she looked up at me again. I guess she was expecting some tears, but I didn't cry. Even as she explained that I would lose every single strand of hair on my body, I didn't flinch.

Up until this day, I still try to figure out how in the world I kept it together. I didn't even feel like breaking down. I didn't feel defeat. I didn't feel fear. It just wasn't present. The decision I made to choose faith over fear had dictated the rest of my plan before it had even taken place…but I had already begin to feel the peace that came with that decision. I take NO credit for that decision. It was not me. I get no glory for that.

The glory belongs to the only wise GOD who decided to hear the prayers, and grant me exactly what I would need to allow HIS glory to be seen. The strength of GOD came in the form of a 37 year old African American single mom, who was about to take cancer by storm!

Michele and I had left the building where I would return in about a month to start my chemotherapy treatments. I didn't know what to expect, but I knew something was coming. It meant the world to me to have my sister there with me.

Her mother was a breast cancer survivor and she had told me if God did if for her mother, she knew He was going to do it for me.

She never cracked under the pressure of the diagnosis. Even in her prayer in the bathroom before we entered the doctor's office...she stated several times "We believe the report of the Lord!"

She kept the faith with me, and told me that I was to speak nothing but victory even in a victim-like state. As we walked to the car, I suddenly felt a tear drop. I was about to lose it. I was about to fall apart. Here it comes.

Just when I was about to give in and fall, something in me stood up and gave me back the strength I needed. Michele looked at me and said "Friend. I'm here. You are going to be fine. We are going to fight this thing. GOD is a healer. You are already fine. Just keep speaking the word!"

Writing this sends me in tears every time, because it was at that moment that I knew, I needed real strength around me because weakness would make an appearance. After all, I was still human. I looked at her and she was serious.

She was so serious! She had one of those looks I had seen before back in High School. Back when I was in the tenth grade a friend had been bullied and she had finally gotten fed up.

She said "I am not playing. She wanna fight? Let's fight!"

After school my friend beat that other girl until she got tired!!! When she looked like she was getting tired, every other girl that the bully tortured began to jump in the fight!

That's the look I was getting from Michele. She was ready to fight until she got tired, and when she did, I would tag in and continue the fight! I said to Michele "I'm here so someone can see GOD. Someone in this place needs to see Him. I'll be fine" With that said, we got in the car and laughed and joked about the blisters she got on her feet from walking in some wedges.

It was the funniest part of the day. We laughed. We laughed in the devil's face. Although I would return to Memorial Sloan Kettering in July to start my chemotherapy, the entire ride home, I laughed with my girlfriend. GOD is good. I was afraid in the natural, but I knew in my heart that God was using me for His Glory and that my story wouldn't end here. It was only beginning.

chapter 2

"Speaking the Word ONLY, Even in the world of medicine"

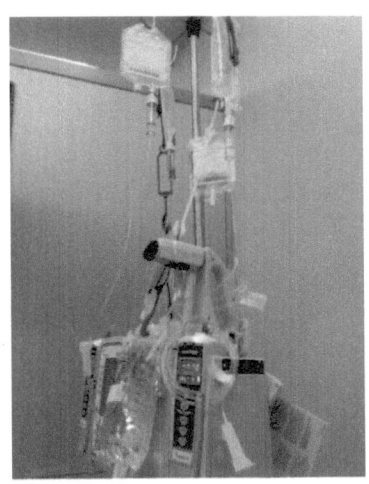

"...but speak the Word only, and my servant shall be healed"
Matthew 8:8

During my "process" I had decided, "I will not say I have breast cancer" which at the time seemed like a small thing. Not knowing that I was actually speaking in to my future.

What I mean by that is, although I was currently diagnosed with breast cancer, and my mouth spoke against it, GOD reached into future time and made it so. Get it?

What I spoke in my "then" became my "now". There were people waiting for me to break down. Waiting for me to "accept" what the doctors said and really "deal" with it.

The problem was I had already accepted what the doctor said...the DOCTOR said it, not GOD. I had already dealt with....it would not be so. See, the thing about cancer, and even doctors of little faith would say... 90% of it is emotional.

Your body responds to certain chemicals that are released when you are happy, at peace, and content.

Those chemicals, called endorphins fight cancer as well. Stress creates an imbalance that feeds cancer cells and makes them stronger. They haven't quite figured out how or why. They have just taken enough "inventory" to watch various patients and their surroundings, and it has always been a better process for those with a good spirit.

Once they shared that with me, I fought hard and long against stress. My job at Verizon was on the verge of going on strike. So what. I didn't care. My health was more important to me.

However, I did check to make sure those health benefits would be in effect, because I'm no fool...good medicinal treatment costs! Let's be clear, because I made certain of my health plan, did in no way shake my faith plan. God ordained some to be doctors, so seeking their help is not going against scripture.

I let life take a detour from drama. I smiled more. I laughed even harder. I cried a little, but I chuckled more.

It's something about being faced with a death sentence that makes you appreciate life so much more.

Things that would have normally stressed me fell by the wayside. People that use to get on my *entire* nervous system couldn't even give me a goose bump. Nary a soul was worth my life. I had to live to tell the goodness of GOD to my child that was watching and for those I didn't even know who I would eventually find out was watching as well.

Life as I knew it had changed. Now knowing good and well that GOD was on my side…I knew that the more I proclaimed life, the more the devil would try and remind me of death. Now to say all was okay all the time would be a lie. I AM human. I am a believer and ALL that, but I am still human.

I am sensitive, I get angry, I get tired, anxious, nervous, fed up; all of these things. Saved and all…those feelings still existed

The only thing that worked in my favor is when I was weak; I had others to bare my infirmities. It's so funny.

Even when I was having not so good days, I would never speak them, I would TEXT it! That's how powerful I believed words were. I wouldn't even SPEAK what my body was going through. After being tested, probed, pulled on, pressed down and tugged at by various doctors, sent here and there, this place and that place, the body has the right to get weary. Sometimes when the body gets weary, so does the mind.

I had a bought with fear, and I had a long bought too. I now view it as; I had to understand the need for courage in order to ask for it. If you don't think you need something right now you might not ask for it, even though there will come a time that it will be needed. I had stored up praise, but I didn't have stored up courage.

I didn't ask for courage, because I was never honest enough with myself to say there was a place of fear.

As I went to these various places for the tests I had to do, I was around people who had the same disease I was diagnosed with, but they didn't look like me, and they didn't sound like me. Would I eventually look like them?

I had experienced a few setbacks during my treatments. I gained a little weight from the steroids that was in my medication. I felt bloated. My emotions became tainted because I was forced into premature menopause which those in that area of life call "chemopause".

I had hot flashes that had me turning on the A/C in October! I had cold spats. Night sweats where I had to just stand in the shower and let the cold water run. It was a trip to drive with me in the winter months. It would be cold outside, but I would have every window down in my car! That wasn't fair to my passengers, but as love would have it, they didn't complain…often. I endured body aches as well. Soreness crept into my lower legs and my feet would ache in the morning as if I walked all night. Things did get hard.

There were days I thought I was being unrealistic saying 'I'm fine', and speaking the Word. It seemed some days that speaking it into existence was more of a fairytale than a non-fiction for me. I did have a moment of anger. It was emotional turmoil to hold my head up and stand strong in weakness, but somehow GOD helped me bare it all.

My service in church was a dancer. Dancing was my passion since I was 5 years old trying to mimic my older brother who was a professional dancer. Every physical joy I experienced in church came through my worship through dance.

I was part of the dance ministry, so the last thing I needed to deal with, were aches and pains in my body. I didn't want my treatments to stop anything I was doing, so I would never speak of my pain. Anytime someone would ask me how I was doing, I'd say "I'm fine! GOD is a healer!" I spoke nothing but the word.

Even when I was having the worse day, full of pain, disappointments, discouragement, and fear…yes fear.

I want to be an encouragement to others. I'm telling you, my go through; it was not what I spoke. I'm not saying it wasn't what I felt. I was not ok, I was in pain. I wanted to quit. I didn't want to dance. I wanted to crawl up in a ball and just wait for the storm to pass. But this soldier wasn't assigned that mission.

Even though my body was riddled with pain, I tried to never ever speak about it. Again, I am human, so I am sure that I had let a few "this hurts!" come out my mouth.

I may have said days later "Oh yeah, my legs *were* killing me!" I would speak in past tense because I had to be very careful with my speech.

With me trying to be superwoman, I had some friendly reminders of certain kryptonite. Still, my cheerleaders were there…. Keeping me grounded.

I have an Aunt that is too a breast cancer survivor and she called every day to make sure I was taking it easy. Even though I wanted to be Wonder Woman, she reminded me that some days I just needed to be 'Diana Prince'.

The cape didn't have to come out every day. Maybe I brought on more pain then I needed to experience by being so bent on not looking sick. That wasn't always a wise decision. Some days, I needed to learn to be still. There was nothing wrong with me not moving just so long as God kept moving.

Going back and forth to my treatments, even in my faith, the mind played tricks even when the spirit was strong. I had wondered if those that were around me knew what I knew. "Speak nothing but the word, by His stripes we are healed" Did they know that even in sickness that they were healed? Did they know that even in this hospital GOD was a miracle worker? I felt sorry for those that didn't. They didn't have the secret, but was that the reason I was here? Was I supposed to tell them the secret? I wasn't sure, but I knew for one thing, nothing but victory would come out my mouth, and anything else? Well, I'll just text the saints and friends and ask them to pray!

As other friends and family found out about my diagnosis, everyone tried to give me their "remedy" for a speedy recovery. A close friend of mine gave me this fantastic little red book of prayers. This book had specific prayers for everything you could imagine, and things you could not.

It was an amazing tool for me. I opened it and searched through it and found a physical healing prayer. It was POWERFUL! It spoke against everything ungodly with such authority and an assuredness! I repeated that prayer EVERY night! I spoke against anything working against my body. I told the devil to beat it! I had things to do for the kingdom and I had my blessing in the flesh to raise. My daughter was only 14 years old. She was not old enough to be without her mom. Death was not an option.

My life almost became a walking confliction. One day I was walking in authority. The next day, I was crawling in defeat. Even as I spoke life, and believed it, I was still human. I had dreams of myself lying in a casket. I dreamed of my funeral often. I didn't understand why GOD would let me see such a thing in my resting hours. It would disturb me to tears. I would get up in the middle of the night and cry. Was I really going to die Lord? Are you showing me my funeral? You know how some people who have gone on said to some that they had seen their funeral and such? I thought that's what GOD was showing me. Showing me how it was going to be. This could NOT be SO!

I remember one of the Sundays that was difficult to get myself together for church. I went to an 8am sisterhood prayer at my church. It was a good prayer, but I had a burden with me. My dreams had disturbed me and shook my faith a little bit. I had come to prayer because I needed to be amongst those who believed GOD with me.

As the prayer ended and I was walking out of the church, one of my sisters came and asked could she talk to me. I didn't mind, so I sat down. She told me she had a dream about me. I was at her house and we were in her bedroom talking. A storm had come and turned everything upside down. Everything was flying around the house, but she and I were okay.

As I sat that, I started to cry because I had just had a conflicting dream last night that I was in a casket. I told her about my dream and she shook her head and smiled. "The 'old' you is dying. GOD is creating a new you. Everything about you will be new".

I started crying so hard. Was it true? Was that what GOD was trying to tell me?

That made so much sense!

I promise you, from that day forth, I had never had another dream about me being in a casket. I received her dream and it became my life. The old me was dying...the new me was coming.

It was coming.

Not here yet.

That was honesty talking, but faith still believing. There were still trials before triumph.

It would be unfair to mislead you and tell you that every day was just sunny and 75 degrees. I had my trials...I had my down days...but with GOD the down days never lasted longer than the upward days. My faith and my walk were strengthened when I acknowledged I had a fear.

I know it doesn't make sense... but the Word of God states in 2 Corinthians 12:9

"My grace is sufficient for you, for my power is made perfect in weakness. Therefore I will boast all the more gladly about my weaknesses so that Christ's power may rest on me."

I spoke that daily. Even if I didn't feel it, I spoke it. Even if some days I didn't believe it, because yes, I dare say it, doubt crept in. It was the enemy's job to make me believe that sickness was unto death.

Every time the fight got hard, I worried a little. I physically felt the drain, but pushing myself to get to church, to be around the saints of God, to be present for the songs, the praise, the preaching. It refueled me. It helped me fight a little longer. I'm careful not to big myself up in this book as I explained the journey, because I was really struggling.

It was hard for me to believe sometimes. As you read some of the paragraphs about me saying this and declaring that sometimes it was through tears, through being laid out on the floor in church crying. Other times it was up and about, with smiles and waving my hands in glee. I remember being so overwhelmed with the drugs in my system that had not yet fully flushed out and I began radiation therapy.

That was my weakest state, and I asked God why me. Why did He choose this for me?

It was too much.

It was too hard.

It was something I did not want to do.

I remember being on the phone just crying after I had text my cousin Tracey about the whys. I remember it like it was yesterday and I still have the text message today. She responded "Why *not* you?"

Exactly.

Why not me? Why didn't God have the right to use who He needed the way He needed for as long as He needed? I was *His* servant. This body was *His* property.

When I drove my car to wherever I wanted to go, it never pulled over and asked me why. When I put the key in the ignition, press the gas, and steered, it went as I commanded it to exactly where I commanded. It went as fast or as slow as I wanted it to go. It stopped when I hit the brakes and it moved when I hit the gas. The only thing I had to do was to make sure the oil was changed on time, the tires were strong, all fluids filled to capacity and the gas tank was full.

I hope you got it.

We are the cars. GOD is the driver. His Word? It steered me. His promise? It fueled me up. His anointing stayed with me, so the oil was always good! And when it got too much? He hit the brakes... let me catch my breather, and then we were off again.

Here's food for thought. There are two types of cars, cars that lose their value with time so they get traded for the newer model, and those that no matter how old they got, they retained their value and become sort after cars, classic cars. I was a classic car and I didn't want to be traded in. I wanted God to use me. I was His car.

The promise of God, John 11:4 kept my tank full! I remained functioning because of it. It is important to understand, without the Word of God being a constant on this journey... I'm not sure I would be where I am today. I'm not saying I wouldn't have survived, because we are all aware that there are indeed godless people who are cancer survivors.

It's in the *'how'* that is so very important. I am a strong believer that my fight with cancer was buffed by God. I experienced a lot, but I also escaped a lot. I am living witness that with God, even chemo had to obey. It was not going to do more than God had allowed it to do. This sickness was real, but it was not unto death, but for the Glory of God that the Son of God may be glorified through it. – John 11:4

chapter 3
The Treatment Plan

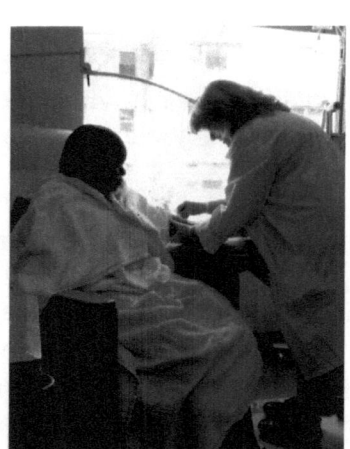

"For my grace is sufficient for thee; for my strength is made perfect in weakness"

2 Corinthians 12:9

Chemotherapy is the treatment for cancer...not the cure. It uses chemical substances to stop the growth of cancer. Sometimes, the treatment can be worse than the disease. It can compromise the body to the point where all you do is sleep and take pain meds. Sometimes it takes away the appetite and if you could eat the ability to hold any food or liquid down.

It discolors your skin, nails, takes your hair, and your strength. It kills ever cell, good and bad. It does not have the ability to differentiate between the two. It was created to kill what had the potential of killing you, but did its own damage on its way.

Many times when you are diagnosed with cancer, the oncologist would offer you to become a part of a trial treatment plan. I had enough trust in my oncologist, so when she proposed the idea of me participating in a new trial...I agreed. I wasn't like a test animal or anything. It was the length of time that was the trial. They wanted to see if giving a specific drug at a different time would have a better effect. Regardless of the timing, the prescription was still chemo, so it didn't bother me to participate.

On my first day of chemotherapy, before they started my treatment, my doctor had explained to me all the side effects that I would have; the blackening of my nails, tongue, possibly skin turning black and being dry, and of course losing my hair. It was I guess a prep talk before the process.

Michele had come with me to my first visit, and my mother had come along. My daughter was away on a much needed vacation, so it was just the three musketeers. As my doctor kept saying what could go wrong, I just kept saying I would be fine. Speak the word only! I believed that. I would be fine. Even though I knew I *would* be fine, I didn't know what to expect, so I was a little nervous.

As the nurse prepared me for my medicine dosage, she took me to a room, with a recliner, two chairs for my mother and 'friendsta' (my nickname for Michele, she was my friend and sister) and free snacks! Yes! I was excited about the free snacks! I was about to have chemo running through my veins, and I was more concerned about getting me a ginger ale and some gram crackers and a sandwich with turkey meat (because I didn't eat pork) all for free. I'm such a ham.

I especially dressed up for this day. I made sure to look like the child of the King. I combed my hair, dressed up and added some fragrance. I was not going to look like what I was about to go through. I refused to look sick.

Once all things were set up, I was giving a warm blanket and a remote. I turned to Law & Order, but apparently, I was told, I was out within five minutes.

Because there was a chance that I had an allergic reaction to the medicines, the doctors prescribed Benadryl in my drip to ward off any allergic reactions and that knocked me completely out! I would have to admit, I enjoyed that. You haven't had a good nap, until you had a Benadryl straight to the vein induced nap! It was good!

When my meds were done, they woke me up and I was on my way. It was just like that. I didn't know what I thought chemotherapy entailed, but it was an i.v to the arm, a blanket and a nap for me. It's amazing how I slept through the process almost every time. I was at ease. Because I was part of a trial… they kept a closer watch on me… took notes on everything and made sure I was at my most comfort level.

Memorial Sloan Kettering had a wonderful nursing staff that I had taken a strong liking to.

Every Thursday I had a different nurse but I greeted them with the same spirit. I would smile, and be just as cute! My outfits, my hair, my smell and my smile let the people around me know, I was different. I might have been in there for what others there had, but I will not respond like others.

Before every session, the nurses would ask me about my side effects.

"Do you have nausea or neuropathy? Had any dizziness or vomiting?"
My answers were always no. When I answered them they would always look and shake their head with a smile.

"You're doing really well!"

No, correction, WE are doing really well. Me and Jesus! Chemotherapy hadn't affected my body as it does others that were going through the exact same treatment
Although no two cancers are ever the same; the treatment plans mimic one another. It's a general rule, chemotherapy for cancer.... But the length and dosage amount is what makes the treatments differ.

I hadn't lost my appetite. In fact, I began to eat any and everything I wanted. I felt if I had chemo in my body, how bad could it be to have a burger? I ate what I wanted, when I wanted, and I slept when I wanted. I lived life to the absolute fullest. I had taken a specific liking to Chef Boy

Ar Dee's Mini Ravioli. I ate it so much, that until this day my mother despises even looking at a can of it. I do too!

I drank my favorite water, smart water, and took my blood pressure pills. I had been afflicted with chemo induced high blood pressure as well. Having blood pressure issues was a minor setback, but a setback nonetheless.

I had to be careful about everything because if my pressure was too high, I could no longer take chemo. So, although I wanted to eat everything in sight, wisdom had me to curb things a bit. I still ate my ravioli, but I just drank a grand amount of Smart Waters daily.

As far as the neuropathy which is the numbness in the fingers and toes I was warned about, it didn't hit in the beginning, so I still went to get my nails and feet done every week.

I did however have to inform my technician to take EXTRA precaution, and sanitary measures, which wasn't much more than what I had already required being that I had a small case of OCD. I had my own utensils that she sterilized every visit and we washed the tub with a special solution before she did my pedicures. It wasn't until my finger nails started turning black that I decided against getting them done. I allowed my body to go through its process without any cosmetic cover up.

I was okay with it because I understood that if people didn't see the go through, they wouldn't believe it. I had to really take completely down and allow GOD's glory to rise. That didn't mean I looked bad per se, but I just didn't cover up my nails because I was trying to hide the blackness. I let my nail beds breathe even if they looked black while doing so.

As I spoke a little about in the previous chapter, I did experience bone pain. My doctor had warned me about it. She said it would feel like I had arthritis. The devil is a liar! Not at 37! I was a dancer too?

I didn't have time for no aches. I fought them tooth and nail. Some days I won…some days it looked like my body won. I would dance every Sunday morning and be in pain every Sunday night. My feet would swell. My legs would cramp. I would cry as my boyfriend tried to massage the Charlie horse in my calf. I still wouldn't give up.

I felt as though, every time I danced for GOD, it was my way of showing Him that I believed He would heal me.

I had sinus headaches because I had lost my nose hairs, so everything went straight up my nose and caused all types of havoc. You never know how important those little pesky things are! Trust me. I do now!

Also, the chemotherapy gave me sinus headaches as well. It was something in the medicine that aggravated the nostrils and caused flare ups of the sinuses.

Great.

Are you kidding me? During my chemo, I had a tooth infection as well. There was no pain like having an infection during chemo. Your body is subjected to so much because your immune system is suppressed. Like I said, I had sinus infections, and then that led to my tooth infection…and well, that led me to the emergency room at 2am, with two drivers that had never driven to the city at night.

God bless my mother and my boyfriend at the time. They tried, but that night, they both worked my nerves! I can laugh about it now, but that night I was so mad at them.

I was laid out in the back seat in incredible pain rocking back and forth and they were asking me for directions.

We've only been to the city a million times. Why did they not know where to go?

After a turnaround or two, The Lord got us there safely, blessed the hands of the doctors to give me some wonderful morphine and antibiotics.

That was my first and last trip to the emergency room during my treatments. I thank GOD for that!

After a few months into my chemotherapy treatment, my oncologist had changed over my treatments to the strongest most concentrated form called Adriamycin. It was part of the plan explained in the beginning by my doctor.

She explained that they were using a clinical trial on me but I needed to do this strong chemo because of the size of the tumor to make sure they get it all. It was only for the four last treatments, but because it was so strong I didn't do it every week. I did it every other week. I went from a medium sized needle of medicine that was accompanied by Benadryl to this Kool-Aid red COLD medicine that came out of the biggest needle you would ever want to see! This medicine is known to former chemo patients as the red devil. It was just that too.

Evil.

I had gone through my other treatments like a champ. Fighting and winning against the side effects and all. I had dressed nice and was jolly to get my treatments started because I looked forward to my good naps and my sandwich and crackers when I woke up.

But after my first treatment of Adriamycin, I realized this was a different type of evil. I cried every other Thursday knowing I had to go get this pain shot up my arm. I cried when I saw the nurse walk in. I tried to mask it. I tried to stay upbeat, but this portion was just really painful. It hurt. It gave me painful side effects.

When the nurses came in, they were covered in what looked like a hazmat uniform. The nurse explained to me that this medicine was so potent that if it touched their skin it would do serious harm. Can you imagine? That was what was going inside my body.

It hurt going in. Imagine if you could, ice cold water going through your veins. If it were possible, it was like brain freeze over my entire body every time it entered. They use to give me warm packs to place on my arm where the needle was inserted but that helped very little.

These sessions took a strong toll over my body. I became weaker, and therefore didn't have the energy to dance. My appetite changed a little. Everything began to taste a little funny to me. Like a metal taste. All but that Chef Boy Ar Dee ravioli and Kum Kau rib tips with barbecue sauce!

Now, I hadn't eaten pork in a month of Sundays, but that meal? I enjoyed the taste of those ribs tips with extra barbecue sauce and shrimp fried rice almost twice a week. I was tired more so I slept more which became a little depressing.

My hormones became more erratic so there were things that I could not control because I was being thrown into a chemically induced hormonally imbalance quickly.

BUT GOD!

I'm telling you, there is something about the go through of the saints that is just different from those that don't know Him! Even as that "red devil" flowed through my veins, it was still no match for the blood of Jesus that flowed through my spirit! Even though it was hard battle to complete, with the prayers of my church family, my Bishop, Pastors and family? I still did not get the worst of it. My nails never fell off like some patients. Only my hands and feet turned black, never my face. I scarred easily, but I also healed easily too.

My body seemed weak, but my spirit man remained strong. I went to church and praised GOD every chance I got! I even mustered up enough energy to give God a dance praise with my feet a few times too! Ran around the church; Stood up, turned around three times, slapped my neighbor, wrote the word HEALING on my tithes envelope and kept it moving with my seltzer water in my little brown paper bag... EVERY SUNDAY!

Eventually, and maybe even finally to the devil's delight, my body began to show signs of a certain go through. I was tired so much. Those last four chemo treatments did it for me.

I couldn't drive myself around that much. I would fall asleep at a light! At this time, I had to stop working all together because I just couldn't do it. I had nights when I asked my mom to just pray over me because I felt my flesh falling into disbelief. I felt like giving up...and just crying defeat.

I remember clearly, waking up to go to the bathroom. I walked in the bathroom and looked in the mirror.

For the first time, I saw the sickness. I saw what cancer had done to me. I saw what it had done to my skin, my hair, my face, and almost my spirit. I cried so hard in that bathroom. I did it silently because I didn't want to wake my mother or my daughter, who was home for the weekend. As I was fighting cancer in my body, I was fighting it in the atmosphere of my life to. As I became weaker, my daughter became more worried and that strained our relationship. She had a hard time processing me living through this.

So imagine, me in the bathroom, crying. Had she woke up to that, that could've shaken her belief in what I told her every day, That it was all going to work out fine. I cried as I took inventory of all. I wish I knew then what I know now. Had I just posted the scripture on the mirror…when I looked at the sickness, and then the Word, I would have probably cried a little less that day.

I do not glorify my go through, nor do I tell the story for pity sake, but I have to highlight it so you can see how far God has brought me in such a short time. Some people battle years with cancer. I was diagnosed officially June 2011, I was officially declared cancer free January 2012!!!

Although it seemed I definitely had 'woe is me' times, God, He never fails.

This is why you have to have the right people around you. The strong bear the infirmities of the weak. If I had weak people around me, who was going to be the bearer?

I was living on my own when I was diagnosed, but with the insistence of my mother, I moved back home so she could watch and make sure I was ok. She didn't want me to worry about rent or anything. Actually, I think it was more for her not to worry.

She felt better as long as she could see me every day. Besides, although my place was beautiful and comfortable and mine, being at home made it easier financially.... one less thing I had to worry about. On some nights where it felt like the cancer was winning, my mother prayed over me.

My child prayed with me and my love prayed for me. I made it through some of the toughest nights of my life, sometimes not being able to even make it upstairs to my bedroom. I slept on the couch in the living room.

Those times, my mother never left me downstairs by myself. As I slept on one couch, she slept on the other. It was like she kept watch for the devil.

Every time I moaned, she started praying. If she wasn't praying, she was reading God's word. I would wake up and she would be sleep, or so I thought. As soon as my foot would hit the floor, she would ask "You ready to eat?"

I thank GOD for my mother. She was very strong during this process. It has to be hard to see your child go through chemotherapy. We had already lost my brother at a young age. I knew she couldn't deal with losing another child, not to a deadly disease. Losing another child period would be too great.

Chemotherapy was hard. It was probably the hardest thing I've ever had to endure in my life. It put me through what is known as "chemopause" which is the term used to describe the side effects of chemo in a woman.

It tricks your body somehow into thinking its going through menopause. So you experience everything that comes with. The hot flashes are the worse! I remember being in my room with the air conditioning on in December! I didn't want to get dressed and I was just not doing well. My treatment left me emotionally and spiritually vulnerable. I was a walking opened wound. It was hard, but we made it through.

Soon enough, twenty sessions of chemotherapy were completed. We completed twenty Thursdays of drinking ginger ale, eating graham crackers, orange juice from Dunkin Donuts, with two glazed donuts & Ramson Allen stealing the Pepsi sodas for the ride home.

It was the grace of GOD that He gave me the hedge of protection in the form of a praying mother, a believing praying daughter, best friends that kept watch and someone who would become, the love of my life.

Chemotherapy kills every cell in your body, whether it is good or bad. I'm thankful it never made it to my spirit. Twenty sessions later, even after the hard last four that nearly broke me, I was still standing.

After the chemotherapy, I had surgery two months later. I had to wait until the chemo flushed out of my system before they would go further in my treatment plan. After the chemo, the breast had shrunk back to its original size. I remember thinking, "Oh great! Now I can keep my breast! PRAISE GOD!"

Again, I went in the office of the breast surgeon fully confident that she was going to tell me that the chemotherapy was enough and I was cured and I could go home.

As I sat there waiting for Dr. Van Zee, the breast surgeon to come in with the good news.

She came in wearing her usual smile. She was pleased with the results of the chemo. So my first words were "Ok so no surgery then right?" She looked at me and patted me on my leg.

"Sweetheart, we still need to take the breast. We have to get that tissue. Conservation is not an option."

I was a little disappointed... but not discouraged. I had been through the ringer with the chemo, so I just wanted to keep the ball going. She explained they would be taking the complete left breast. Leaving me with two options, to have reconstruction done, which would add four additional surgeries, or live without a breast. I chose to go the full Monty and opt for reconstruction.

January 4, I had a full left mastectomy of the left breast. Since I chose the option of reconstruction, an expander was put in my chest at the time of removal. The job of the expander was to stretch my skin in preparation for reconstruction.

After eight weeks of healing time, I began the radiation treatment part. Every day for five weeks I had to endure beams and high levels of x-ray type treatment to kill any "left behind" minuscule cancer cells. Radiation hurt. It burned and it took my energy. It was hard to get up every day. It caused fatigue and I didn't want to do it.

I remember one visit as I was sitting to be called in for my treatment, a man walked in for his treatment. His neck was red and he had a white cup in his hand. He walked slowly and he seemed to be just more exhausted if not more than I was. He was alone and just as he approached the chairs, he fell to his knees. His energy completely left him. As the nurses ran to help him up, he just said "I can't today. I can't do it. I can't. I'm so tired. I can't stand."

As I watched this man, I thought... I was here with my family. I was tired but I walked in on my own. I was tired but I was able to stand. I was low on energy, but I still was able to move about. A tear fell down my face. Not sure if it was for that man or for me....but when they called my name, I hopped up, went in, changed my clothes and got my treatment.

At this time, my hair was in full bloom and I had a head full of curls making out a little cute afro. The technicians complimented me on my hair and told me that I looked pretty. I felt ugly, but I appreciated their kindness.

Cancer is horrible... but like I said, sometimes the treatment is just as bad or worse. However, God still gave me grace. My skin that was radiated... did burn, but my doctor suggest that I use an ointment called Aquafore after every treatment and drink insane amounts of water and I would be fine. I'm here to tell you, that is exactly what helped.

I prayed every time I applied the ointment. Didn't matter what the doctors said, if it wasn't God ordained, it wasn't going to work. I'm grateful that every treatment worked in my favor. Even through the pain, I was supplied grace. I was told of my strength.... But I never thought I was strong. I just felt like I was doing what had to be done so that God could get the glory.

There were days I felt like I was just going to fail God because of my wrong responses. I was not always in the best spirits. This process was longer than what *I* bargained for. I thought I was going to have an immediate healing because *I* said so. I didn't see the bigger picture like most of us don't. I look back now and get it, but I didn't then.

After my five weeks of radiation, it was time for my next step.

Expanding.

This was the process where the skin was stretched to form a breast replacement. It was uncomfortable, but quick. They inserted water into the surgically placed pocket in my chest and it stretched my skin. Once it was the desired size, it was time for the tram surgery. June 2012, I underwent a major surgery, where I had a fat transfer from my stomach to create a breast. Yes. They do that. Amazing isn't it? They removed fat from my stomach, tucked the stomach, rearrange the blood vessel to supply blood to the newly formed breast and created an areola.

Without getting any more graphic, it was lot of reconstruction of my abdominal wall. In fact, there is a muscle that was moved that causes my rib cage to protrude on the left a little further than it dos on the right. It used to bother me, but compared to what I've been through, that's a very minute thing to notice.

I've had chemotherapy, radiation, and reconstruction that involved four major surgeries.

I stand here, naturally *and* spiritually reconstructed. I certainly don't look like what I've been though. You would only know these things because I've told them. My surgeries and their results are all undetectable. That skin that was burned during radiation has returned to its normal color.

The feeling they said I would lose in my underarm after my mastectomy surgery? I feel everything. The feeling they said I wouldn't have in the place where they built me a breast? I feel. The only set back I may have is because of the change in muscle structure, I get Charlie horses in the left breast often! The muscle that used to support my abdomen now formed the breast, so it's like a stomach cramp in the breast.

It catches me off guard and it's hard to explain to people why I'm getting a Charlie horse in my breast without going into detail. After this book, I hope to never have to explain that again!

My body has been diagnosed, deconstructed, reconstructed and even after had a few setbacks, but I am a firm believer that my attitude of hope and faith is what helped me push through. It is important to believe the outcome will be in your favor.

The scripture that stuck out the most at this time was "my grace is sufficient"

And it was. God granted me grace to continue. His grace kept me in spite of my desire to want to give up, and give in. He sent the right people, the right doctors, the right Word and I was made whole. I will forever give Him glory AND credit for my survival.

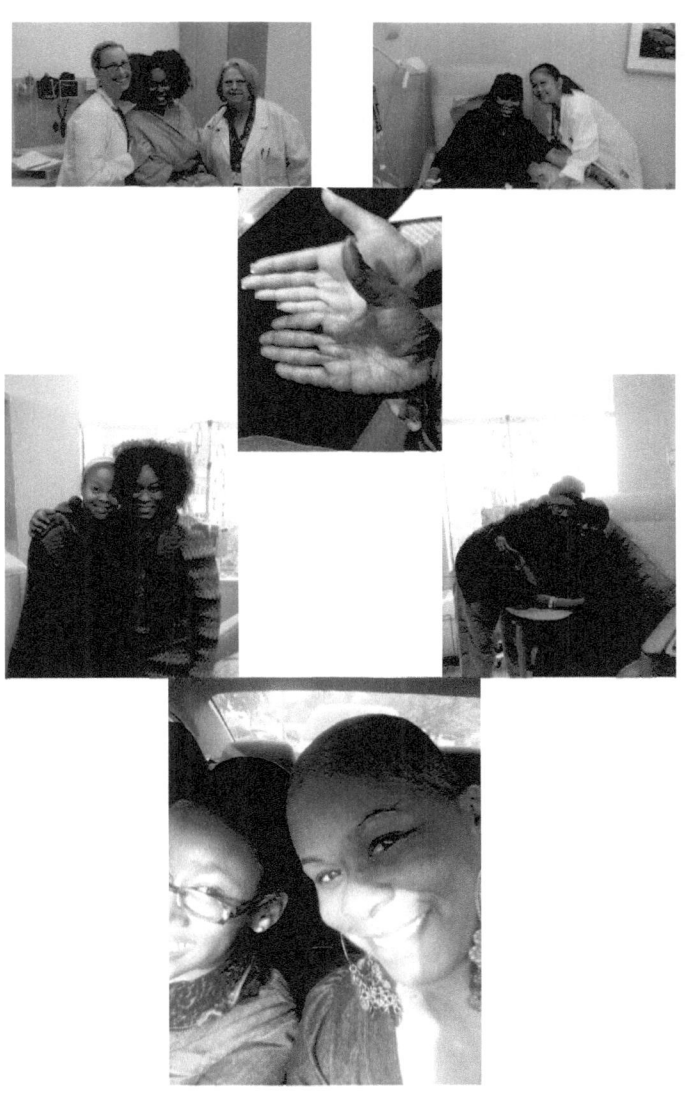

chapter 4
The Fading 'glory'

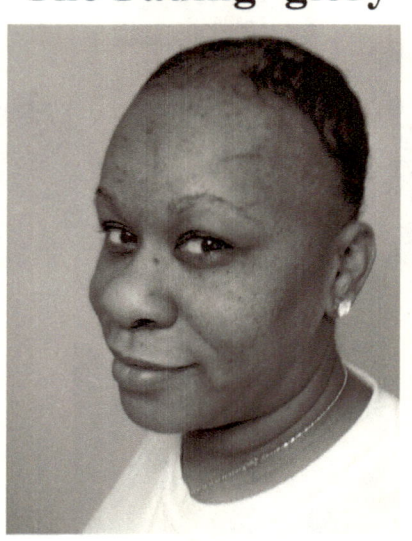

"…for long hair is given to her as a covering…"

1 Corinthians 11:15

All women love hair. Whether they were born with it or bought it. It's our glory. It's our pride and our prize.

That's why the hair industry is so lucrative because we love hair. I was blessed to have a head full of thick, healthy long black hair. I cut it at will, because it grew back in a week or two. I colored it different shades, put braids in, took braids out, and wore it curly, but mostly straight. I had hair all of my life.

I never *needed* a wig, and never wore a wig. The most I added to my hair were synthetic box braids. My hair was my joy. My Bishop use to tell me he liked to see me dance because my hair would be swinging. I loved my hair. I loved my hair. I loved my hair. And it almost broke me to lose my hair.

I will never forget, when the doctor told me my hair would fall out, I believed God to allow that 'cup' to pass me. I wanted to do His will, but I wanted my hair while doing it. I was born with a head full of hair. I have never been bald. My hair has been my beauty affirmation for all of my thirty seven years.

I will never forget. I noticed a little shedding coming around my third week of chemo. I would run my fingers through my hair and a little more than a strand would be in my hand. I still had more hair on my head than in my hand so I didn't pay it much attention. I still believed that maybe, just maybe, God would allow me to keep my hair.

I pulled my hair up into a ponytail figuring if I didn't comb it, the hair would stay in place; Silly woman.

One night I was in the bathroom combing my hair and out of nowhere a big handful of hair just came out. I looked at the comb and looked at my scalp. You couldn't tell because I had really thick hair. So I figured okay, I can hide the thinning parts. But one more stroke proved that this was more than thinning. My hair was simply falling out rapidly.

It was coming out and it was coming out in bulks. As any woman would do, I cried. I don't care if you were sitting on the right hand of GOD! If your hair fell out on the streets of gold, you would not be doing good!

That day was probably the most hurtful and disappointing days. I called for my mother because I was just standing there holding in my hands hair that was supposed to be on my head. I was standing there with almost my faith falling in the sink with my hair.

My hope was falling. Everything was leaving me because I was so sure that this one thing would not come upon me.

I called for my mother. It was a distress call. The kind that it doesn't matter where you are, or what you were doing, if your child cries out, you're there.

My mother calmly walked up the stairs to the bathroom. She almost seemed unbothered. She looked at me and looked in the sink and then back up at me. She said "Well, I guess the medicine is working. So it's time to cut the rest off"

She rubbed my back and walked back downstairs. I stood there a little longer, and I did cry. I looked in the mirror and realized, I was about to physically change. People would now be able to see what I was going through. What was I going to do without my hair? Who would I be pretty to without my hair?

I was stripped of the very thing that I perhaps held high. My hair was a form of a GOD to me and God was not into sharing glory. He needed me to be completely submitted to this journey. He needed people to see what I was trying to hide. It's amazing. I didn't want to be bald because I felt then people would show pity and then I would become the 'sick girl with no hair'.

It's sad how I put so much weight on my hair being my safety net, but it was. It hid me from a lot of things.

I looked back in the mirror and repeated the words my mother said, "The medicine is working. That's why my hair is falling out. Ok. Time to move on

Again, I wasn't invincible, I had moments, but they were short moments I believe because of my relationship with God. He never left me and at this time in my life, He wasn't quiet either. I called one of my girlfriends who did hair and told her I needed my hair cut down. I went over to her house and she cut what was left of my hair into the cutest low yet still feminine cut.

That lasted all about a week, because the hair kept coming out.

I ended up going to my cousin who was a barber and he cut it all off.

Going through trying not look how I felt, I discovered something. There weren't many options for ethnic women when it came to wigs, make up and scarf choices. At the hospital, they had a store with many options from scarves to head pieces and they even gave you recommendations to go to a certain salon to purchase your "medical headpiece" better known to most of us as a good ol' wig! I was devastated when I went to the place to get my "prescription". All the wigs in the store looked like fake hair.

They looked plastic and they did not represent me at all. I never had long silky plastic looking hair. I never had thick auburn bangs that lay across my face like little strings of thread. I wanted my type of hair back on my head. My texture. My hair.

One day, one of my sisters from my church, took me to a wig store. She showed me how to choose different colors and styles. She encouraged me to have fun with it. Since I had to wear a wig, choose a color that I never wore before. She encouraged me to try new things and new styles. I remember trying on all types of wigs that complimented my skin tone, Fun wigs with big curls and not so big curls. It was in an ethnic friendly neighborhood, so the choices were more to my kind of style.

I picked up a tri colored wig that had some loose curls to it and I felt confident. I was ready to go! Once I got over the initial hump of wearing a wig, I went to the stores on my own looking for my "signature" look.

I remember the first time seeing 'Erin' on a mannequin. She was a big jet black curly afro.

I loved it.

I didn't even try it on in the store. I purchased it and went home excited about trying on my new look. Suffice to say, 'Erin' was my go to wig every day for three months. Yes. You read correctly. I was bald for only three months. My last chemo treatment was on November, and by February at my girlfriend's wedding, I had my hair. It was baby fine and just a dusting over my head, but it was my hair and it was on its way back

During my times of being without hair, my confidence level was threatened. I wore scarves to the best of my ability, but they were hot on my head and I didn't like them too much. I couldn't always wear the wig unfortunately, because another side effect of the treatment was having extremely sensitive skin. So the lace front of the wing irritated me sometimes. It even caused scarring. Sometimes, I had to settle for the scarf.

One Sunday, the dancers had to dance with praise and worship. I was trying to fix my scarf so it wouldn't come off while I danced. I was in the mirror getting frustrated with it and the leader of the team (My angel, Angelique) came in the bathroom.
"Fancy Pants, take that off. Let the people see your head. Stop hiding. Stop fighting. You're beautiful. Let it go."
Angelique probably doesn't know this, but she changed my perspective that day.
'Let the people see'
Hiding what I thought the devil was doing *to* my life....I became so busy covering and trying to hide what God was doing *in* my life. If they didn't see me bald, would they ever believe I lost all of my hair and it came back? If they didn't see the go through, what was the point? God needed me to stop resisting and release my hold on hiding.

I took the scarf off and walk out to the front of the church bare. I was bare not only without my scarf, but without a concern in the world. I didn't care. I was battling for my life and vanity didn't have one weapon to help me in this fight so there was no need for it to be present in the battle.
As Angelique began to sing I looked at her and she winked and smiled. When she began to sing, I danced and

it was such a relief. I was free. I let God do whatever He wanted to however he wanted. I didn't care what anyone said. Yes, when I walked out I heard the gasps, I heard the "omg, she's sick" "Oh her hair is gone" I heard it all. I just didn't listen. I danced my way into another victory that day. Praise and Worship was particularly powerful that day too.

Angelique held me up spiritually and that gave me a natural strength.

When praise and worship was over, and I was in the hallway, Angelique came out and prayed with me and covered me. We cried and cried. We probably would have still been there crying had not a young lady from the church come and hug me. Her words,
"Thank you for being brave. I never thought I would see anyone that was like me"
She pulled back her wig and revealed that she too had lost her hair, but was too ashamed to tell anyone. She said she was thankful that I allowed God to use me. It gave her strength.

I was floored, humbled, and even embarrassed. I was so busy trying to cover up the process that I was hindering the progress.
God wanted that Sunday to happen exactly the way it did. The only reason why someone saw me in a wig ever again wasn't from shame of being bald, but because I really just loved the wig and being that I was still subject to getting sick all the time, I needed a covering on my scalp and that scarf was never an option. It was just too hot.
I was not as strong as I hoped I would be when my hair fell out, but I wasn't as weak as the devil hoped either. There were times where I was more carnal than spiritual, more vain than necessary and it all taught me.

My good, my bad, and even my indifferent moments have all pushed me into an area of sensitivity that I did not have before. This hair loss journey was less about the chemo and more about my sisters. There are women in this world that struggle with baldness going through treatments for numerous things, but we sometimes never know. However, we may laugh or comment about their wig choice, their hair style or anything. I'm in a different space now. I can chuckle at someone's hair, but God quickly reminds me....

'Francys, you never know what someone is going through, or what it took for them to get out of the house, just like you when you lost your hair so be mindful.'

I'm thankful for my growth during my journey, and daily I begin to understand more and more why things happened the way they did.. I am also here to tell you that every strand has returned to my head better than ever. It grows even faster now. I am natural of course because the state of my hair was just better left to its own. When my hair grew back I did however take advantage of it being short, by, uh, kind of keeping it short. It grew in nicely... and quickly, but I kept it trimmed to a style that I might not have otherwise been bold enough to achieve having to cut all of my hair off. When my hair grew back I took advantage of it being natural and short and became more experimental with color. I was so happy to try new things I wasn't necessarily bold enough to do before. One time I colored my hair bright red.

My Pastor told me I looked like Woody Wood Pecker.

He even asked Ram why he allowed me to do that to myself.

That was funny.

Then, I shaved one side of it. I was so excited to try new things that I did so much to it, but however, I have regained my senses and I am letting the glory grow as long as it wants to. No more scissors and definitely no more clippers. Maybe a little color here and there, but I'm thankful, my "covering glory" has returned.

chapter 5
Assignment Revealed and Assumed

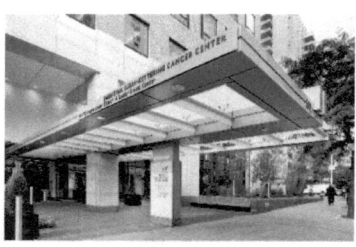

... "God of all comfort, who comforts us in all our tribulation that we may be able to comfort those who are in any trouble, with the comfort with which we ourselves are comforted by God"
2 Corinthians 1:4

Breast Cancer and its treatments consumed my daily life. Everything I did or said had something to do with it; whether it was the doctors or people asking me why I was wearing a wig. It had taken a life of its own. I didn't understand at first why it happened.

But after much prayer and quiet time with GOD I understood more and more daily that it was never about me or my body, but the GLORY that GOD needed to get and where He needed to get it from. I learned that whatever GOD's will is, it's perfect, and it's acceptable.

I also learned, whatever He wants done, its going to get done with or without you. There was someone that needed to see my strength derived from GOD and that person would first be me. It wouldn't be until I got to my weakest point that I would realize my strength.

Going through with the cancer, everything around me seemed to shatter. My job was getting on my nerves about time taken off time for treatment, my daughter wasn't handling the fact that her mom was going through chemo, thus she started acting out and misbehaving.

My seemingly cool and calm functioning relationship with her dad had gone with the wind, and my family members were getting on my nerves about silly fights.

It just seemed that at this time in my life everyone would just calm down right? Everyone would notice that I had been diagnosed with breast cancer and the foolishness would stop right? Please. Just as sure as there is a GOD there is a devil and he wasted no time getting busy.

I had developed great relationships with all the staff at Memorial Sloan Kettering. My nurses, doctors, technicians; Even the cleaning crew. Everybody loved the girl who smiled every time she came for her treatment.

When they all asked how I was doing, I would always say "I'm blessed" And they would respond "You certainly are" Confirmation. That's all I needed was for someone to agree with me. I had some good days and not so good days, but I was always blessed. On one appointment, my oncologist, Dr. McArthur asked me how I felt about talking to another patient who wasn't dealing with her diagnosis too well. She said whatever it was that was getting me through this, that I needed to share it. All I could think of was ok yep this is it! Assignment!

So I signed up for my "assignment" and met a beautiful girl who was just as scared as I was, just as concerned as I was, and just as young as I was.
Her mom loved my hair and asked how long it took to grow back.

Once I revealed that it was one of my favorite wigs, they both just looked astonished. I told them, it's about finding what works for you and having fun with it. Try looks you would never try before. I gave the advice I was given by my gem, Lady Regina Harris.
The young lady, who was Caucasian instantly became my "pink" friend. She came to visit me while I was in chemo. She said she needed to see me immediately to talk about her treatments.

She walked in to my chemo suite, and although that particular day wasn't a good one for me, I wore my smile, and asked God if it was HIS will, give me the strength to not put on a front but put on my faith. Let my faith precede my current situation before I open my mouth.
As I began to speak with her, I promise you, I began to feel better.

My sinuses eased up a bit. My smile became genuine and I was ready to be the example God needed for this young lady. She and I became text buddies.

My mother and her mother became instant buddies as well.

I have a charm hanging from my rear view mirror still to this day that was made for me by new friend's mother.

She made my mother a bird pillow adorned with the breast cancer ribbons. They were a sweet family that became family. We kept in touch as much as possible and would keep each other up to date with treatments and surgeries. My mother and I shared the goodness of God and the grace that kept us during this process. It was an opportunity to show how even through this God was still a good God.

About a month after meeting her, my oncologist came to me and gave me the biggest hug.

She said she didn't know what I did, but whatever it was, it helped her and her patient get off the rocky road and start the healing process.

As I sat on the bed after my hug and exam, I only wanted to do one of two things, give God the biggest hug, and cry.

How selfish have I been all my life not to have ever come here on my free will and tell about the goodness of Jesus? It never crossed my mind to really come visit the women at the breast center.

However, as quickly as that thought left my mind, I had another God induced thought....

"It's better received while you are going through it. They can see me in you while the cancer is in you too!

I would tell you that that was my one and only assignment, but that would not be true. I was assigned to many people suffering with cancer...... and they weren't all physical either. I began to read the scripture about being a living epistle.

God needed the healed to tell of His goodness everywhere. The doctors needed to know that unless Christ is in the medical plan, there is no need for a medical plan.

Now, let me be clear, I am not saying there is no survival for those who do not know Christ.

How silly would that be?

How many people do you know that are in the world and have beat cancer? I know PLENTY! However, what I am saying is... my journey through it WITH HIM is NOTHING like it is without Him.

I will not believe it is as easy, as caring, and as protected without Him. No amount of money or fame can give you the peace you get from spiritual nepotism. My daddy took care of His daughter!

I had family members that had changed their hearts toward God after seeing what I went through and how I went through it. When they heard I had cancer, many of them prepared in their hearts for the worse, because that's what they felt that word was synonymous with.

I had to fight through a lot of things, not for myself but for those that were watching.

That was my assignment during this ordeal. To allow the manifestation of healing take place right before their eyes. The tricky thing was that I had to be sick. I had to have rough days. I had to have rough nights. I had to go through. My daughter had to gain a little fear for me to see the greater need for faith.

My one and only child, when I was going through had a rough time. When I was writing this book, I had asked her how she felt about me telling what went on between us.

At the time of me writing this book, she was away in college, so I sent a text. You know those college students don't answer their phones much. When she responded, I decided, instead of my words, I would use her words, the exact way she said them, because it was her true feeling.

Below is a text message that summed up our journey together through the disease.

The Pink Purpose   My Story for His Glory

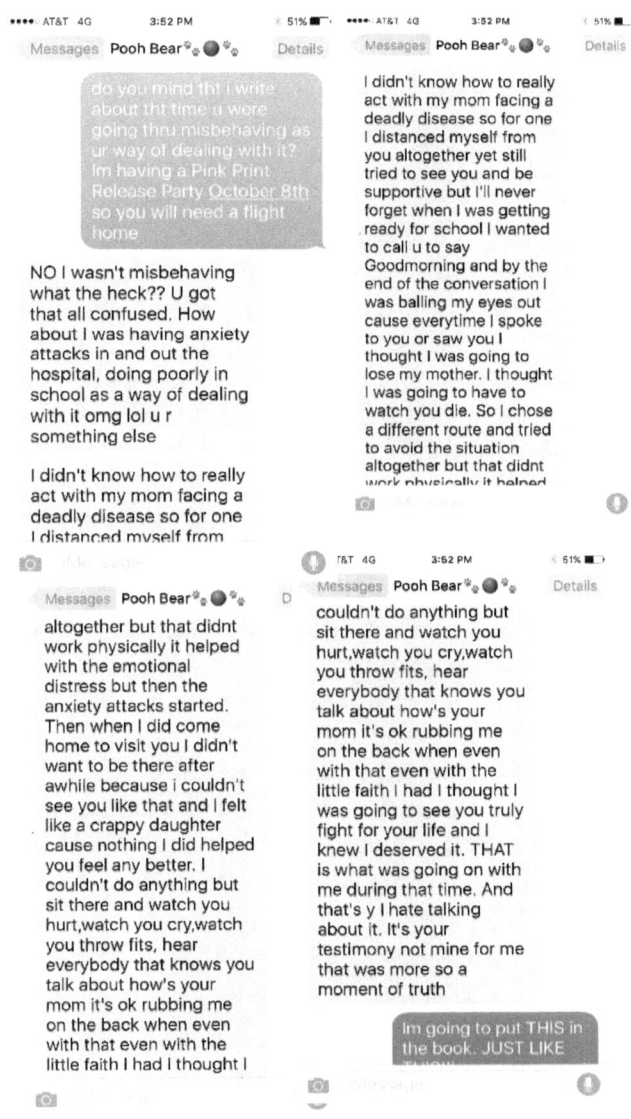

75

My daughter and I don't talk much about it and it makes her uncomfortable to see pictures of me when I was sick. I was blessed to have her father be able to take over the complete load while I was sick. She stayed with him and he made sure she got to and from school, breakfast, dinners, laundry and basically life with Daddy while I was healing.

She doesn't like to refer to that time much, but what she does love to see, are the walks we do every October in Central Park. The sweatshirt I wear that says "SURVIVOR". She likes to see me playing in my hair. She likes to see me trying on clothes talking about how great my new boobs look in them. My assignment wasn't only for strangers, but it was for someone right at home. My mini me.

I was challenged to live out the things I sang about, prayed about and encouraged her to do the same. I had to not only talk about Jesus, I had to live Jesus....and make Him famous through it. Every decision, every response... I had not only an audience outside of the home, but I had a domestic one too. I'm not too sure if I made every single correct decision.... But I am certain that my daughter has seen firsthand the power of God manifested....and for that.... It was all worth it. Every pain, every strand of hair lost....every surgery.... For the Glory of God to be exemplified.....it was worth it. A charge to keep I have... and a God to glorify!

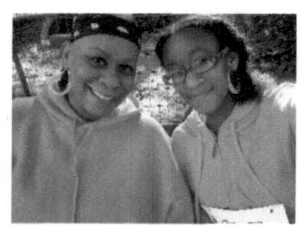

As I was finishing up this book, I was given another assignment. I will never forget being asked to speak with one of the Pastor's wives at my church. The church had given her a "GAVE CANCER THE BOOT" party and I was honored to be a part of the celebration. She really did give it the boot!

With so much style and grace, never missing a beat!

I remember being invited to the party as a surprise guest. The night before as I was gathering my stuff to dance, I came across my sash that I got the first time I did the cancer walk in central park. I held onto it as a souvenir and kept it nicely folded. As I looked at it and God spoke right then and there. He told me that this thing that I kept as a souvenir was really a torch and I needed to pass it along.

The sash said SURVIVOR.

I packed it along with my dance clothes and after I danced, I gave her the sash. It was a torch that she will pass along to the next survivor and the next will pass it on. I said all of this to say... I did not survive to be a "souvenir"... I survived to be a torch; to pass along the goodness of His healing power. That is why I had to go through the COMPLETE fight. My assignments are still being assigned. I take them all as they come because I am the torch. One thing I want to leave with you, there is a time to hold on to things... and then there is a time to pass it along. Make sure you know the difference between a souvenir and a torch.

chapter 6
'Common cold, not so common'

*"**Wisdom is the principal thing; therefore get wisdom; and with all thy getting get understanding.**"*
Proverbs 4:7

This is probably the shortest chapter in the book, but still necessary. As a cancer patient, as a believer in Christ… sometimes I didn't follow the orders of the doctor. That wasn't wise.

I put my faith in motion but didn't use wisdom. I will never forget, when my Bishop prayed over me, he instructed me to believe AND do what the doctor says.
I did half of it for a quick minute.
I had faith that everything was going to be okay but I didn't take the necessary precautions to make it a little easier on the journey. It is important as believers to understand that taking medicine does not dim your faith.
Taking chemotherapy does not make you a weaker Christian. In the Bible, scripture says, that WISDOM is the principle thing! Wisdom must be applied in all things.
During chemotherapy, the doctors made sure to tell me not to be around too many sick people, after chemotherapy, they advised me not to do so much because my body had to rest. During radiation, they advised me to sleep as much as my body wanted. After my surgeries, to rest and not lift, not to walk a lot up and down stairs and not drive long distances. I mentioned those instances because every single one of those things I ignored and I paid dearly for them.

I will start with during chemotherapy.

I was told I would get tired and to let me body rest. So I did the complete opposite. I ran, and ran. I went to this house and went to that restaurant.

I went anywhere my car would take me, and because of that, I brought on fatigue faster and stronger.

Had I listened to the doctors and took it easy, maybe those nights I crashed and burned wouldn't have come so often.

During radiation my body was exhausted, but I insisted on not missing a church service.

As if God couldn't be wherever I was, I went to church one time too many without proper rest and when I got home, my body gave out. I couldn't walk, I couldn't sleep and I cried. I felt defeated. Not because God wasn't healing me, but I wasn't allowing the healing to take place. I was too busy running away from the acknowledgment that I needed to, well sit down.

After my mastectomy, I was told not to lift anything heavy. With mastectomies comes the chance of having lymphedema, the retention of water in an affected limb. So what did I do? I went grocery shopping. Lifted the bags and ended up in the hospital for a lymphedema flare up.

I still now deal with lymphedema flare ups. My left arm pains me so bad sometimes it requires prescribed medication.

It swells up sometimes that I can't even put a shirt on over it. I have to wear a medically prescribed compression sleeve and gauntlet whenever I drive long distances or fly.

I live for Lycra and stretch cotton now. Most of my coats that I loved I can no longer wear because it is tight on my left arm. Had I listened to the doctors and did what I was supposed to do, perhaps my arm wouldn't have been subjected to lymphedema. I'm not complaining that I have it, because I'm still here, alive and well. It's just that, some things could have been avoided.

Also, my diet needed changing and I didn't change it right away. My immune system was compromised from chemotherapy and it is said that your immune system will never fully return to the strength it had prior so you have to work on eating the right things, and exercising. Doctors also told me to watch my stress levels. The immune system is affected with stress levels too.

Well, again, I didn't heed to instruction. And because of that, my immune system wasn't strong enough to fight off the shingles.

I had the shingles in the worse part of my body, the arm that had lymphedema. It was a painful experience and I had to be hospitalized for ten days to get the needed medicines in my body quickly which meant intravenously.

My veins haven't made a full recovery as of yet since chemo, so they had to do a PICC line (an intravenous line threaded through the vein until the end is near your heart) That PICC line was uncomfortable going in. I experienced an unnecessary and perhaps an avoidable pain.

I promised God that when I got out of there I would take even better care of my body and treat it as the temple He saved. I have given up pork for good. I don't eat beef, chicken finds its way on my plate on the rarest occasions and turkey is my treat.

I am trying to change over to becoming a pescetarian, in which my diet will mostly consists of veggies and fish. Now, as a woman of color, growing up on chicken was a birth right. Fried, barbequed, smothered, baked, and well fried. It's unfortunate that we are not knowledgeable of the harmful things we put in our bodies. The intake of chicken excessively is not good for anyone but especially women. Hormones in chicken mimic the hormones that women naturally have.

The fattest parts of the chicken have the most hormones and with industries wanted faster and fatter birds, they inject antibiotics. It's too many things that can go wrong with the mixing of hormones so I'm not really interested in eating chicken.

There is no need for me to eat any chicken breast plumped up to a double D. Too much. It will confuse my own hormones and have them fighting against each other, causing cells to activate cancerous.

The fast food today is not conducive with healthy living. I don't think it ever was, but everything is in a rush.... So we grab something quick and heavy and not realize our body is being deteriorated just as quick. It is not in the best interest of anyone to have a diet of sugar, artificially colored drinks, candy, manipulated meats (sandwich packaged meats) empty caloric foods without necessary nutrients.

We do not work out as much as we should. There is not enough walking, drinking water and full resting taking place. Our body needs these four major components to be healthy, healthy diet, rest, water, and exercise.

It is important that while you want God to heal your body, listen to the instructions that the doctor gives.

Remember, Luke was a doctor, the beloved doctor Pray that God gives you the discernment when to receive

instructions and when not. Hearing instructions from a doctor during your healing process is not receiving his report. We believe the report of the Lord! Always! Pray for wisdom, to know what to do and what not to do, because sometimes, God's will and the doctor's advice line up! I recently watched this show on Netflix called "What the Health" and it has given me information that I need to pass on. There are so many links to animal consumption by humans and sickness. Processed meats contain so many contaminants. Chickens are being fed all type of antibiotics. Pigs are being fed pigs!

I'm not here as a proponent for the vegan diets. I am a firm believer that what we pray over to eat is indeed blessed.

However, I do want to say, we must monitor the consumption amounts of foods that are not made to feed our health more than it is to just fill our bellies. I miss the days of seeing my uncle grow his own vegetables and it was garden to table for me as a young child. I think if we go back to perhaps having more fresh vegetables, grains and fruits in our diet, more live food than dead flesh on our plates…we can avoid a lot of sickness in our bodies.

chapter 7
"Pure Love"

"Love is patient, love is kind. It does not envy, it does not boast, it is not proud. It does not dishonor others, it is not self-seeking, it is not easily angered, it keeps no record of wrongs. Love does not delight in evil but rejoices with the truth. It always protects, always trusts, always hopes, always perseveres. Love never fails…."
1 Corinthians 13:4-8

You know, when you are looking for love, you find everything but. It's something about that unexpected appearance made by love. It was June 2011, two weeks after my diagnosis.

My Bishop was being installed into Presiding Prelate of the Pentecostal Churches of Jesus Christ. I took the bus from Brooklyn to Connecticut to celebrate his installation. I had nothing on my mind but survival. I had dealt with the fact that I would be starting chemotherapy in a month and I would move on with my life. I was single and not looking.

The guy that I was interested in, when he found out about my diagnosis, he told me that he did not want to continue even getting to know me much less consider dating me because he had known too many people that died from it and figured I had just a matter of time. That had not only closed my heart up, but locked it and gave God the key. His words almost frazzled me, but I was still cute! I just believed what I believed and after deleting him from my life, I was not looking for anyone else to disappoint me or challenge my belief; especially not now.

I had too much on my plate. I however was happy. I just believed GOD was doing wonders, and because of that, I didn't walk around with the sad face. So it was nothing to me that as I walked around from the offering during the service to have this gentleman smile and wave at me, and for me to smile and wave back. I went to my seat and thought nothing of it.

We had an evening service that same day, and as fate would have it, I sat in the same row as the man who waved at me at the morning service.

He was nice.

He was funny...and he was cute!

We talked generically about the services as I turned back and forth trying to avoid another man who sat next to me with his legs so wide, that his knee was touching my leg. Can you say uncomfortable?

I began to try to figure out how to remedy my discomfort and came up with the idea to switch seats with my daughter. My daughter and her friend were smaller than I was so I asked them to switch seats with me.

Neither would.

However, there was a vacant seat next to the nice guy who waved at me earlier, who somehow ended up in my row. I ended up sitting next to him, and well I could say the rest is Allen history, but GOD wouldn't get the glory from that short story…so let me tell it. I was not at all interested in getting to know anyone at this point in my life; Especially having had to deal previously with someone who definitely mishandled the situation as my 'suitor'.

I was dealing with the fight of my life and I needed no distractions, but it was something about him.

That night, we laughed and talked as much as we could during service and it felt like I was laughing with an old friend.

We became quick friends and soon feelings followed. It hadn't been three weeks later that I had to tell him what I was dealing with. He asked me out on a Thursday, but I couldn't go because I had a doctor's appointment. I remember Ram asking me where my appointment was. Thought that was weird, but just figured he was nosey. Yes. He *was* nosey.

I thought about not telling him. I still felt a way. On one hand.. I didn't know him well enough to tell him that much of my personal business and that was indeed personal… and honestly, I didn't want to lose the new fun that had entered my life. But a calming came at the thought of sharing the news with him.

However, I didn't verbalize it. I sent him a text telling him what hospital I had to go to hoping he come to his own conclusion. After the text, we never really spoke about it again. He didn't even respond past an "Ok"

I was for certain that he was a goner. You see, I expected the same outcome from this guy as I had from the previous one.

Well, God had something else in mind.

It was a Tuesday night after church, and he and I were talking, just idle chit chat. We somehow got back on the subject of the Thursday date.

He said to me, he had to cancel his request because he was busy. He had to go with a friend to the doctor as well.

Nope, didn't connect the dots there either.

We continued to talk and eventually, he just came out and said "you're the friend I'm going with. I want to be there" I remember this like it was yesterday.

My first words "Boy don't play with me. I don't need to be getting attached to you right now. I have enough going on."

His response..verbatim.. "But what if I'm already attached to you?"

I guess that's it in a nutshell. From that day on, we became attached. Every day he was there for me. Every appointment he was there for me. He listened to the doctor as they explained to him the rough road ahead and he never flinched. I would give him credit, but GOD was all up and through there. It wasn't our plan at all to get together.

He wasn't looking for anything, and neither was I.

However God was. He was looking for two people that would come together and make Him the center of their relationship. I had previous relationships, but my needs were the center of them and his flesh was the center of his.

Not this one. It would be one that was tried and true, spiritual, emotional and fruitful. Ramson and I became a couple at the lowest point of my life. What I used to attract and keep men in prior relationships, I no longer had. My beautiful hair had all fell out; my body was not an option, because it belonged to GOD.

My smile wasn't always present because I was in pain, and my cute feet and hands were blackened.

All I had to offer him was my heart. It was just as fragile, but that's all I had to give. The great thing about it, that that was all he had to give to. So, we exchanged hearts and promised to take care of them like they were ours.

Through every mood swing and crying spell, I had my boyfriend right there. He mastered the art of ignoring me when I was being extra, paying attention when I was being quiet. Praying with me was important. I had never prayed with anyone I was in love with. That's probably why the other relationships never worked.

But, with Ramson, prayer was the core. We prayed at the hospital, we prayed at home, and we praised in church! It wasn't always an easy relationship, we had break ups, make ups, walk outs, walk back ins. It was a lot. We were fighting each other at times we were supposed to be fighting the devil. All in all, our hearts meant God.

We meant GOD together!

Ram and I became the best of friends.

I remember the day my hair fell out. I was in the bathroom wrapping it so I could cook. (I didn't like to cook with my hair out)

I took one stroke and all of the hair just fell in the sink. I froze. This could not be. So I put the brush down and combed it. More hair in the sink. I put the comb down and ran my fingers through my hair only to have my hand full of hair.

It was coming out and it was coming out in bulks. As any woman would do, I cried. I remember, Ram was watching TV and I guess he heard me cry. After my mother left the bathroom, Ram came to the door and said
"So what! You still fine with no hair!"

He kissed me and walked away like I wasn't standing there with my hair in my hands. I looked back in the mirror and repeated the words my mother said, "The medicine is working…"

When I went to the barber to cut the last of my hair off Ram was right there smiling. He never made me feel any less beautiful than I did the first day I met him with my head full of hair.
He complimented my eyes and my smile and told me I was so pretty. What was great was he didn't just tell me with his mouth. The way he looked at me every day told me too. God had placed a good man in my life for me to continue to feel like the woman I should even if I felt I was at my lowest point.
My emotions had us in arguments and disagreements often, but Ramson knew it was the medication and its side effects.
Still, he had every right to walk away because I was not exactly the easiest to get along with. His patience was golden. Nothing short of Boaz potential!

He and my mother got along great and my daughter grew to love him and trust him because of the way he took care of me.

When my daughter went away on vacation, she said to me "If Ram's there I'm okay. I know he'll take care of you"

As I said before, my daughter had been dealing with the diagnosis a little hard, as to be expected, but Ram eased tensions with her too. It was an all-around blessing.

I didn't look up one day, and didn't see his face or hear his voice. When it was time to have my mastectomy, I felt some kind of way, but in his own little way, he made me feel confident that life would only get better after this. And it did. After chemotherapy, after five surgeries, expansions, radiation, and just life itself, Ramson Allen stayed, and asked me to stay as well.

On November 18, 2013 he asked me to be his wife and we were married September 13, 2014.

God thought enough of me to give me a great man to love me for the only thing he needed to love me for; my heart, my intention for GOD and my obedience to follow Christ. I thank God for that. joy and happiness played a big role in my smiles every day. There are days that we are better at this marriage thing than others, but that's ANY marriage and can happen at any time, because that's just life.

Two imperfect humans trying to do a 'perfected' thing...... becoming one. When I look back over my journey with him, and I see what we've already come through together? It's no doubt that I married my best friend with all of his flaws and he married his with all of hers and if we beat cancer together, we can beat anything together!

chapter 8
LIFE AFTER LESSONS…..

The first thing I've learned in my survivorship is that all survivors handle life after differently. Having gone through such a traumatic, life altering experience, it's hard to blame others in how they handle their "life after". I'm thankful I've had the chance to understand the different survivors… it has helped me help them.

Before I really prayed for understanding, I use to get almost offended by those that didn't want to talk about having beat cancer. I didn't understand why they didn't want the world to know how strong they were. Or annoyed by the survivor who went right back to giving in to their vices without regard to their bodies being compromised. It almost made me angry

Then there was the fearful survivor, who lived in constant question if the disease would return. I've watched someone become so consumed with "what ifs" that they missed the 'right nows'.

She is getting better at just living and not going over her life trying to figure out or pin point the exact moment she did something that caused her cells to activate cancerously.

I found myself being the "A Typical" survivor; the survivor that would tell the world my story.

I would show off my reconstruction without hesitation and share all the details of my journey, because not only was I thankful to still be alive, I was amazed at all the handy work that went on. I was beyond impressed by God. I went through a deadly disease, but didn't suffer like most.

I didn't lose my nails like most women do during chemo. Yes they turned black, but that was it. It was almost like God left the gate open wide enough for the devil to put his toe in but never allowed him full access to me.

Surviving cancer is a constant journey.

Sometimes a memory will take you back to a place of worry, or an injury would give you extra concern. Life is never exactly how it was before. It is nearly impossible. For some of us, we carry around permanent "beauty marks" across our chest where our breasts use to be. I can be transparent. I was hospitalized in June 2017 twice for an infection from a mosquito bite on my compromised arm. The first time… I was in a room by myself and all was well until they took me upstairs where other patients were.

There, for the first time in a long time… I lost it. I cried! I begged them to take me home because I wasn't sick and I didn't even want to see anything that would remind me of from whence I came. I didn't know that thing was still in me. As I type this I shake my head at the memory of how I felt; the reminder that there still was a little unhealed wound that I didn't fix because I didn't face it. The nurses pleaded with me to stay to take my medicine because it was important to get ahead of the infection.

My husband pleaded, my daughter pleaded. I stayed, but on the condition that they took me back downstairs into the area where it was just me and no one else. It was called the "Decision Unit" where the rooms were a little secluded… everyone had their own room, closed off pretty much from the rest of the hospital world.

They obliged me and I was taken back downstairs….given the needed medicine and sent home the next morning.

However, the conviction that followed was terrible.

Between that and my husband saying "you never know babe, maybe there was someone that needed to just see your face". No way did I want to receive that. I was like….I'm good. Still though, the conviction sat on my chest like a brick. I repented and I told God if he ever wanted me to meet someone I would do it. I wouldn't fight it. Guess what? Not seven days later... I was bit again and I was back in the hospital. They told me they had to keep me to get the antibiotics in quickly. I didn't fight it. I said ok... and two things happened. I met a wonderful lady who was my neighbor in the room. She had just had lung surgery and they found no cancer! Thank God! She wanted to know why I was there. When I told her, she praised God. We talked about being cancer free and she said she was nervous and scared but after she saw me walking around she was ok. How about that! I was there not only for that but for me.

I was there to face that fear demon and to conquer it. If I had to be there, God was there.

Simple.

He would not send me somewhere He had not already been and prepared my hedge.

I stay dint he hospital two nights and two days... and I walked the floor I was on thanking God for His healing power and asking Him to walk with me and touch those that was on that floor. I asked Him to give whoever needed peace, strength, healing, faith and love. I repented for allowing fear to creep up. I am healed. I am whole and I have to work daily to make sure the devil knows, he has no room in my headspace or my heart space to plant any seeds! I do not want sickness to come upon me to go see about the sick. I ask God daily to help me prioritize my schedules, and finances to do what I was definitely called to do and that is to speak about His COMPLETE healing power!

To unveil that, and still smile, is strength. I applaud each and every survivor.... the gun ho survivor, the ignorant survivor, the fearful survivor, the careless survivor, and the survivor who feels unworthy.

The one who doesn't know God personally, but understands His power and wonders why or how he could care enough about them to heal their bodies. It's amazing how vastly wide the spectrum of survivors is. There is someone in your life right now, surviving from something.

It may not be cancer, maybe not of the body, but it can be cancer in the mind or in the heart. Once you know what kind of survivor you're dealing with.....you can learn and apply the best love. That's all we need.

Survival is still a fight; a fight against your own will and to understand that everything was done on purpose... in purpose.

It is very important for people dealing with survivors to understand what category they fall in. You can better help them knowing their perspective. You may not agree, but it's their way of dealing with it.

Not everyone is strong enough to remember, record, write, and relive that part of their life enough for someone else to understand. It opens them up to a level of vulnerability that only another survivor could understand.

I am a survivor who feared just a little, but had more faith, a survivor who cried, but prayed.... Who even worried for a second, but believed. It is human nature to be human.

We are flawed... and it's ok. It is however, our greatest growth in life to see our flaw and not just accept it, but seek the other side of it, the remedy of it... and in that seeking; it always leads us back to the Faultless, Flawless One. God.

There wasn't a chapter specified or dedicated to, but I want to take this time to talk about and appreciate the caregivers of those going through it; you matter. You make the difference

You are needed and most importantly wanted. As I think about every time my mother had to sleep on the couch, my daughter had to bring me water, my boyfriend had to figure out my taste buds for the day....friends tip toeing around my chemo induced menopause mood swings....There will never be a day that I feel like I can say thank you enough. You are the lifeline to your loved ones. You may think that there is nothing you can do, but by simply being present encourages the heart. Even if it's hard on you, it's harder on them. Be there. Be there. Even if it's just to stare in the eyes and say "you can beat this" be there. Any human's emotional and physical strength can flourish in an atmosphere cultivated by love.

My fellow survivors from not just breast cancer, but any cancer, any deadly disease for that matter; There are many things that will go through your mind when sickness hits. Thoughts that it's your fault, you did something wrong, God is punishing you, or the exact opposite...you will know God wants to get the glory.

Whichever is your immediate....you must know in all things to give God thanks. My journey happened the way my journey was supposed to. I pray that you all are encouraged in knowing that God is the author and the finisher of our fate. I believe my most important component in my journey was the foundation of hope and faith, secured and built daily by attending services weekly... sometimes two or three times. It was important that during my physical weakness that I tried to keep the spirit strong.

There is enough negativity in this world that can sour your spirit... so it is important to have a spiritual foundation. You will need it.

God has everything under control and His plan has the perfect ending.
I wrote this book as a testimony. With all the obituaries stating that this one and that one passed from cancer.... I had to write my story to let people know, I went through cancer. It was not easy. It was life challenging, but it was also life changing. It connected me with people and it also disconnected me with people.
My gains outweighed my losses.... But my losses were still mourned. I am human.
I experienced a serious sickness. It was a growing process and sometimes growth comes with pain. Any survivor from cancer will tell you, aches and pains are never regular anymore. What you deem as a basic headache, for a cancer survivor? Cause for concern, your mind plays tricks with you, wonders if came back in another spot. Calls the doctor to tell them you have a pain and may need an MRI. Those are panic requests. When the doctor wants to do more tests on you, or calls you to redo tests.
Panic sets in.

That is a fearful way of living. I have to plead the blood over my mind every time I'm not feeling well. The devil will not get another shot at me. I am healed. This is a hard journey...However, it was a necessity and where I am at now?
I can say, I can finally say, I appreciate what I went through. This journey has opened new doors for me. There are doors that lead to peace for you too. There is one thing

that stays with me, even after my journey through the sickness ended and I want to share with you.

I noticed a need for more resources for ethnic women suffering from the disease. We do not deposit enough in our own communities so there are no resources to pull from like those in other "ethnic races". We must pull together and make certain that the same opportunities are available across the board.

We are in need of beauty company donations, hair and wig donations, or referrals. There is a need… and with my foundation **Glow in Pink**, we will make it our best to fill the gap. I chose the name **Glow In Pink**, firstly because when you think of the word GLOW … you think positive thoughts, you think beauty, you think strength, power. Pink, you think feminine, soft, and now, because of its commonality, breast cancer. Together, I want to translate the vision of STRENGTH even through a sickness for patients. I want to encourage empowerment during the fight; glowing beauty, for …well the ashes. For those suffering from any form of cancer, your story may not be like mine and it may not end up like mine, but there is GODLY victory in every story if He gets the glory. Don't let man take the credit. It is all the doings of the Lord that we grace this earth, healthy happy and whole. Nothing works unless He allows it.

The weapon (sickness) may indeed form, but it will not prosper. Again… that is not the will of the Lord. With that being said, live out His will for your life.

       Live it as God himself would have you to.
       Get proper rest,
       Eat well.
       Exercise often.
       Laugh more.
       Develop a personal relationship with God

Not just when you want Him, but let Him know He's always needed. God is not a genie and His job is not to grant us three wishes, but if we walk up right before Him he will give us the desires of our heart. If we walk up right, our desires become His will, and of course He will always bless us within His will.

I cannot give Him enough credit. It was by His grace that I am cancer free. My latest test results from my survivorship program states that my body shows no evidence of cancer ever being present. There is no residue. There is nothing but a 'beauty mark' across the left man made breast. It is not my scar.

God gave me beauty for ashes and I bless him for it. This book, I hope it blesses you. I hope it encourages you. I pray that my transparency into my journey helps you to understand that there is always a purposeful plan after the pain.

Thank you for coming with me as I reconnected with my journey. It wasn't easy. The memories weren't always pleasing, but the pain never outweighed the plan. God kept me. I thank Him for it. To someone who may be going through this trial, please know…. Your words are powerful. You have the power to command the atmosphere to be in your favor. Speak to your body and command it to obey the Word. It is to be in good health.

**My name is Francys Renee, the DancinWriter, the daughter, the mother, the sister, the wife, the SURVIVOR...
and I'm Pink on *and* in purpose!**

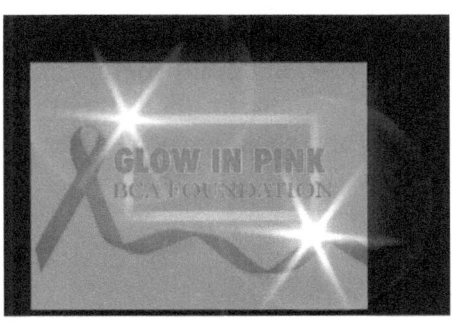

**For more information contact
Francys Renee
for more personal assistance you can email her
@
iglowtoo@yahoo.com
or
thedancinwriter@yahoo.com**

Francys Renee, the wife, the mother, and the daughter, the sister, is also known as the DancinWriter. Her 'brand' is giving ode to her God given talents and gifts of dance and writing is a breast cancer survivor.

She is an author of two Christian Fiction books with her debut novel entitled 'The First Lady', and its sequel 'Deceitful Hope'. 'The Pink Purpose' is her first non-fiction book release for her publishing company Suite 74.

Suite 74 is a "multi-room" entertainment group which is home for many in the gifts of dance, mass media and print works and spoken word artists.

Dedicated to all of my pink fighters, pink survivors and… …To the angels who got their wings…glowing in pink.

I love you.

www.ingramcontent.com/pod-product-compliance
Lightning Source LLC
Chambersburg PA
CBHW021437170526
45164CB00001B/274